ESSENTIALS OF NEURAL SCIENCE AND BEHAVIOR

Study Guide & Practice Problems

Ronald Calabrese
Department of Biology
Emory University

James Gordon
Director, Program and Physical Therapy
New York Medical College

Robert Hawkins
Center for Neurobiology and Behavior
College of Physicians and Surgeons of Columbia University

Ning Qian
Center for Neurobiology and Behavior
College of Physicians and Surgeons of Columbia University

APPLETON & LANGE
STAMFORD, CONNECTICUT

Front Cover: A photomicrograph of a section through the primary somatosensory cortex in the rat. Inputs originating from the thalamus have been labeled with a red florescent dye. These thalamic fibers form dense groups of synaptic terminals in layer 4 of the cortex. Each separate bundle of fibers relays information originating from a single large whisker on the animal's face, and forms the basis of an information-processing column of cortical neurons. The array of these columns forms an orderly representation of the animal's face in the cortex. Photomicrograph by Alejandro Peinado (Albert Einstein College of Medicine) and Lawrence C. Katz (Duke University Medical Center).

Prentice Hall International (UK) Limited, *London*
Prentice Hall of Australia Pty. Limited, *Sydney*
Prentice Hall Canada, Inc., *Toronto*
Prentice Hall Hispanoamericana, S.A., *Mexico*
Prentice Hall of India Private Limited, *New Delhi*
Prentice Hall of Japan, Inc., *Tokyo*
Simon & Schuster Asia Pte. Ltd., *Singapore*
Editora Prentice Hall do Brasil Ltda., *Rio de Janeiro*
Prentice Hall, *Englewood Cliffs, New Jersey*

ISBN 0-8385-2221-1

Acquisitions Editor: John Dolan
Production Editor: Todd Miller
Designer: Elizabeth Schmitz

PRINTED IN THE UNITED STATES OF AMERICA

ISBN 0-8385-2221-1

9 780838 522219   90000

Contents

Symbols

C Capacitance (measured in farads).

C_{in} Total input capacitance of a cell.

c_m Capacitance per unit length of membrane cylinder.

E Equilibrium (or Nernst) potential of an ion species, e.g., E_{Na}.

F Faraday's constant (9.65×10^{-4} coulombs per mole).

G Conductance (measured in siemens).

g Conductance of a population of ion channels to an ion species, e.g., g_{Na}.

g_l Resting (leakage) conductance; total conductance of a population of resting (leakage) ion channels.

I Current (measured in amperes). The flow of charge per unit time, $\Delta Q/\Delta t$. Ohm's law, $I = V \cdot G$, states that current flowing through a conductor (G) is directly proportional to the potential difference (V) imposed across it.

I_c Capacitive current; the current that changes the charge distribution on the lipid bilayer.

I_i Ionic current; the resistive current that flows through ion channels.

I_l Leakage current; the current flowing through a population of resting ion channels.

I_m Total current crossing the cell membrane.

i Current flowing through a single ion channel.

Q Excess positive or negative charge on each side of a capacitor (measured in coulombs).

R Gas constant (1.99 cal $\cdot$ K^1 $\cdot$ mol^1).

R Resistance (measured in ohms). The reciprocal of conductance, $1/G$.

R_{in} Total input resistance of a cell.

R_m Specific resistance of a unit area of membrane (measured in $\Omega \cdot cm^2$).

r Resistance of a single ion channel.

r_a Axial resistance of the cytoplasmic core of an axon, per unit length (measured in Ω/cm).

r_m Membrane resistance, per unit length (measured in $\Omega \cdot cm$).

V_m Membrane potential, $V = Q/C_{in}$ (measured in volts).

V_R Resting membrane potential.

V_T Threshold of membrane potential above which the neuron generates an action potential.

V_{in} Potential on the inside of the cell membrane.

V_{out} Potential on the outside of the cell membrane.

Z Valence.

γ Conductance of a single ion channel to an ion species, e.g., γ_{Na}

λ Cell membrane length constant (typical values 0.1 – 1.0 mm).

τ Cell membrane time constant; the product of resistance and capacitance of the membrane (typical values 1 – 20 ms).

Units of Measurement

A   Ampere, measure of electric current (SI base unit). One ampere of current represents the movement of 1 coulomb of charge per second.

Å   Ångström, measure of length (10^{-10} m, non-SI unit).

C   Coulomb, measure of quantity of electricity, electric charge (expressed in SI base units s · A).

F   Farad, measure of capacitance (expressed in SI base units $m^{-2} \cdot kg^{-1} \cdot s^4 \cdot A^2$).

Hz   Hertz, measure of frequency (expressed in SI units s^{-1}).

M   Molar, measure of concentration of a solution (moles of solute per liter of solution).

mol   Mole, measure of amount of substance (SI base unit).

mol wt   Molecular weight.

S   Siemens, measure of conductance (expressed in SI base units $m^{-2} \cdot kg^{-1} \cdot s^3 \cdot A^2$).

V   Volt, measure of electric potential, electromotive force (expressed in SI base units $m^{-2} \cdot kg \cdot s^{-3} \cdot A^{-1}$). One volt is the energy required to move 1 coulomb a distance of 1 meter against a force of 1 newton. Measurements in cells are in the range of millivolts (mV).

Ω   Ohm, measure of electric resistance (expressed in SI base units $m^{-2} \cdot kg \cdot s^{-3} \cdot A^{-2}$).

Preface

This workbook is intended as a companion study guide to *Essentials of Neural Science and Behavior*. The questions in the workbook follow the text closely. After completing the chapter in the textbook, students should immediately attempt the True/False Questions, Completion Problems, and Matching Problems. These are designed to reinforce key points in the textbook and do not necessarily represent typical examination questions.

The Synthetic Questions and Quantitative Problems are more in the nature of examination questions. These questions sometimes go beyond the textbook and require synthesizing ideas from more than one chapter and thinking beyond the facts. The model answers to these questions and problems should be studied carefully. Finally, some problems in the chapters that deal with cellular electrophysiology (Chapters 8 through 11) are specifically designed to give students the benefits of practical experimental work using the NeuralSim computer simulation programs provided with the textbook. NeuralSim includes two simulation programs: APSIM simulates the action potential and passive electrophysiologic properties of an axon, while PSPSIM simulates excitatory and inhibitory postsynaptic potentials.

Students who consistently use the workbook together with the textbook should find the study of neural science easier, and more rewarding.

Brain, Nerve Cells, and Behavior

Overview

In Chapter 1 the evidence for the localization of function in the cerebral hemispheres is reviewed by focusing on the historical development of our understanding of the neural bases of language. We have come to realize that, like all behaviors and cognitive functions, language is the product of the interaction of discrete brain areas that represent elementary neural operations and which are interconnected by serial and parallel pathways. Language function is also lateralized, being localized in the left hemisphere, which controls the right body side. The left hemisphere is considered dominant in most people as it controls the right hand, which is likewise usually dominant, as well as language. Functional specialization of different cortical areas is associated with cytological differences between these areas. Each area contains an orderly sensory or motor map of the body, depending on its function.

Modern techniques like PET scanning, which can be used to observe the physiological correlates of behavior in active human subjects, confirm the idea that different aspects of language are localized in a number of discrete areas that interact through serial and parallel pathways.

In Chapter 2 of the text the nervous system is viewed from a different perspective — from the cellular connectionist point of view. The simple monosynaptic stretch reflex is explored as a way of understanding how neuronal properties and synaptic connections form functional neural circuits that produce behavior. Cellular connectionism is based on the tenets

1

of Ramón y Cajal, specifically the principles of dynamic polarization and connectional specificity. The first of these principles is best summed up in the words of Cajal: "Every neuron possesses a receptor apparatus, the body and dendritic propagations, an apparatus of emission, the axon, and an apparatus for distribution, the terminal arborization of the nerve fiber." (We now realize, however, that some of these elements may be missing or merged in some neurons.) The second of these principles may be summed up as follows. Neurons make specific connections with particular targets at specialized points of contact called synapses, and this specificity endows neural networks with their functional capabilities. The monosynaptic component of the stretch reflex illustrates these principles of organization and the various signals and signal transformations that neurons use to communicate.

When a muscle is stretched, activating muscle spindles, the amplitude and duration of the stretch is reflected in the graded amplitude and duration of the receptor potential in sensory neurons of the spindles. If the receptor potential exceeds the threshold for action potentials in the sensory neurons, the graded receptor potential is transformed at the neuron's trigger zone into a train of all-or-none action potentials, which continue as long as the threshold is exceeded. The larger the amplitude of the receptor potential, the higher the frequency of action potentials; likewise, the longer the duration of the receptor potential, the longer the train of action potential continues. The action potentials are conducted into the spinal cord without failure or attenuation

At the presynaptic terminals of the sensory neurons in the spinal cord, the frequency of action potentials determines the amount of transmitter released onto the postsynaptic motor neurons. The released transmitter, by interacting with postsynaptic receptors, determines the amplitude of the resulting excitatory synaptic potential(s) in the motor neuron. The graded synaptic potentials spread from the dendrites to the trigger zone at the axon hillock, and there, if they exceed threshold, they initiate action potentials. These action potentials are then conducted without failure or attenuation to the terminals of the motor neurons on the muscle. There, they initiate transmitter release and thus produce excitatory synaptic potentials in the muscle, which trigger action potentials in the muscle fibers and cause muscle contraction. Thus, a simple stimulus initiates a simple movement, the knee jerk.

Objectives

1. Understanding the historical development of our current view of the localization of function in the cerebral hemispheres.

2. Understanding the principles of cellular connectionism, illustrated by the stretch reflex.

3. Understanding the various signals and signal transformations that neurons use to communicate.

▦ MATCHING PROBLEMS — PERSONS

1. Neuron doctrine

2. Phrenology

3. Aggregate field view

4. Cellular connectionism

5. Mass action

6. Cytoarchitectonics

7. Language dominance of the left cerebral hemisphere

A. Pierre Flourens

B. Carl Wernicke

C. Franz Joseph Gall

D. Pierre Paul Broca

E. Korbinian Brodmann

F. Camillo Golgi and Ramón y Cajal

G. Karl Lashley

■ MATCHING PROBLEMS — CONCEPTS

1. Receptive aphasia

2. Expressive aphasia

3. Conduction aphasia

5. Distributed processing

6. Serial and parallel processing

7. Elementary brain operations

A. Left

B. Processing of the different components of a single behavior

C. Processing in a discrete local region

E. Wernicke's area

F. Processing in all sensory and motor pathways

G. Arcuate fasciculus

■ COMPLETION PROBLEMS

1. There are two distinct classes of cells in the nervous system: _____ and _____.

2. A typical neuron has four morphologically defined regions: _____, _____, _____, and _____.

3. Most neurons have only one axon but several _____.

4. The cell body (_____) is the _____ of a neuron; the dendrites serve as the site for _____ to a neuron; the _____ is the main conducting element of a neuron, and the _____ are the output elements of a neuron.

5. The information conveyed by an action potential is determined not by the _____ of the signal, but by the _____ of the signal.

6. Many axons are surrounded by a fatty insulating sheath called _____, which is interrupted at regular intervals at _____, where the _____ becomes regenerated.

7. The space between a presynaptic terminal and the postsynaptic cell is called the _____.

8. The number of processes is a useful way of classifying neuronal types into three large groups: _____, _____, and _____.

9. Neurons can be classified functionally into three groups: _____ (or _____), motor, and _____.

10. Interneurons are of two types: _____ interneurons and _____ (or _____) interneurons.

11. There are three main types of glial cells in the vertebrate nervous system: _____ and _____, which form _____ in the central nervous system and peripheral nervous system, respectively, and _____, which are the most numerous and have several functions.

12. The connections between sensory and motor neurons in the monosynaptic stretch reflex circuit illustrate both _____, in which each afferent neuron synapses on several motor neurons, and _____, in which each motor neuron receives synapses from several afferents.

13. Neurons typically produce four types of signals at different sites within the cell: an _____ (receptive) signal, _____ (trigger) signal, a _____ signal, and an _____ (secretory) signal. This functional model of the neuron embodies the principle of _____, put forth by Ramón y Cajal.

■ TRUE/FALSE QUESTIONS

(If false, explain why)

1. The speed of conduction of action potentials in mammalian axons is between 0.1 and 1 m/s. _____

2. The size of axons in mammals ranges from 0.2 to 20 mm in diameter and from 0.1 mm to 2 m in length. _____

3. In most vertebrate neurons the axon hillock acts as the site where action potentials are initiated in response to synaptic inputs to the dendrites and cell body. _____

4. The neuron doctrine set forth by Ramón y Cajal holds that neurons are the basic signaling units of the nervous system and that each neuron is a discrete cell, whose several processes arise from its cell body. _____

5. The principles of dynamic polarization and of connectional specificity, while useful in the time of Ramón y Cajal, are not thought to apply to neurons and neural networks today. _____

6. Multipolar neurons predominate in the nervous systems of invertebrates. _____

7. The sensory neurons of the dorsal root ganglia of vertebrates are pseudo-unipolar. _____

8. In most neurons there is a negative correlation between the number and extent of dendrites and the number of synaptic inputs the cell receives. _____

9. There are between 10 and 50 times more neurons than glial cells in the nervous systems of vertebrates. _____

10. Glial cells are supporting elements, produce myelin, scavenge debris, buffer external K^+ ions, guide the migration of neurons during development, form the blood-brain barrier, and nourish nerve cells, but they do not participate directly in neural signaling and information processing. _____

11. In monosynaptic reflex circuits the sensory and motor neurons have one layer of interneurons interposed between them. _____

12. The afferent fiber from a stretch-sensitive muscle spindle has its cell body in a dorsal root ganglion and projects a central axon into the spinal cord. _____

13. Stretching a muscle activates several hundred sensory neurons, each of which makes synaptic contact with 100 to 150 motor neurons. _____

14. Afferent fibers from muscle spindles make synaptic contacts with projection interneurons in the spinal cord that transmit information about muscle length to higher regions in the brain. _____

15. In neurons hyperpolarization is excitatory and depolarization is inhibitory. _____

16. A reduction in the membrane potential of a neuron to a more positive value (about 10 mV) can initiate an action potential. _____

17. Receptor potentials and synaptic potentials are local signals that spread passively from their site of origin and thus attenuate sharply over a distance of 1 to 2 mm. _____

18. Receptor potentials and synaptic potentials (input signals) are graded in amplitude, but action potentials are all-or-none. _____

19. In mammals action potentials are about 100 mV in amplitude, 1 ms in duration, and travel at speeds of up to 100 m/s. _____

20. The intensity of sensation and the force and speed of movement is determined by the frequency of action potentials in a sensory or motor neuron, while the duration of sensation or movement is determined by the period of action potential production. _____

21. The message of an action potential is determined entirely by its temporal relation to other action potentials in the same pathway and not by the pathway itself. _____

22. Feedback inhibition enhances the effect of an active pathway by suppressing the activity in competing pathways. _____

23. Functional diversity among neurons results from diversity at the macromolecular level, and thus results from differences in gene expression. _____

24. Orderly synaptic connections among groups of neurons make it possible for relatively simple and uniform neuronal components of the nervous system to process complex information. _____

SYNTHETIC QUESTIONS AND QUANTITATIVE PROBLEMS

1. Identify the major areas of the left cerebral cortex involved in language.

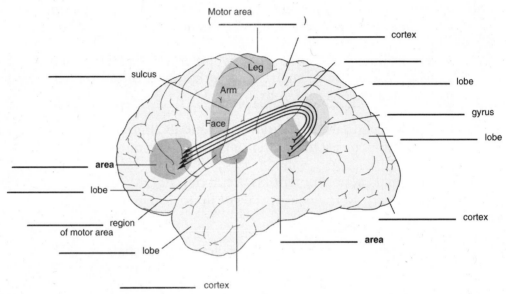

Figure 1–1

2. Identify the four signaling components of neurons and the type of signal produced by each component.

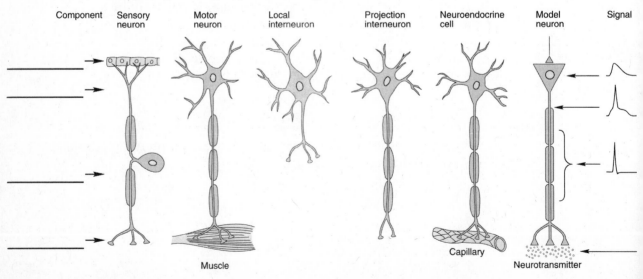

Figure 1–2

3. Fill in the appropriate range of values for each type of signal.

	Amplitude	Duration
Local Signals		
Receptor potentials		
Synaptic potentials		
Propagated Signals		
Action potentials		

Answers

▨ *MATCHING PROBLEMS — PERSONS*

1. F.

2. C.

3. A.

4. B.

5. G.

6. E.

7. D.

▨ *MATCHING PROBLEMS — CONCEPTS*

1. E.

2. D.

3. G.

4. A.

5. B.

6. F.

7. C.

COMPLETION PROBLEMS

1. neurons; glia

2. cell body; dendrites; axon; presynaptic terminals

3. dendrites

4. soma; metabolic center; synaptic input; axon; presynaptic terminals

5. form; path

6. myelin; nodes of Ranvier; action potential

7. synaptic cleft

8. unipolar; bipolar; multipolar

9. sensory; afferent; interneuronal

10. local; relay; projection

11. oligodendrocytes; Schwann cells; myelin; astrocytes

12. divergence; convergence

13. input; integrative; conductive; output; dynamic polarization

■ TRUE/FALSE QUESTIONS

1. False. The speed of conduction of action potentials in mammalian axons is between 1 and 100 m/s.

2. True

3. True

4. True

5. False. The principles of dynamic polarization and of connectional specificity, proposed by Ramón y Cajal, are *still useful* in understanding neurons and neural networks.

6. False. *Unipolar* neurons predominate in the nervous systems of invertebrates.

7. True

8. False. In most neurons there is a *positive* correlation between the number and extent of dendrites and the number of synaptic inputs the cell receives.

9. False. There are between 10 and 50 times more glial cells than neurons in the nervous systems of vertebrates.

10. True

11. False. In monosynaptic reflex circuits sensory and motor neurons make direct synaptic connections; *no interneurons* are interposed between them.

12. True

13. True

14. True

15. False. In neurons depolarizations are excitatory and hyperpolarizations are inhibitory.

16. True

17. True

18. True

19. True

20. True

21. False. The message of an action potential is determined entirely by the neural pathway in which it is carried.

22. False. *Feed-forward* inhibition enhances the effect of an active pathway by suppressing the activity in competing pathways.

23. True

24. True

SYNTHETIC QUESTIONS AND QUANTITATIVE PROBLEMS

1.

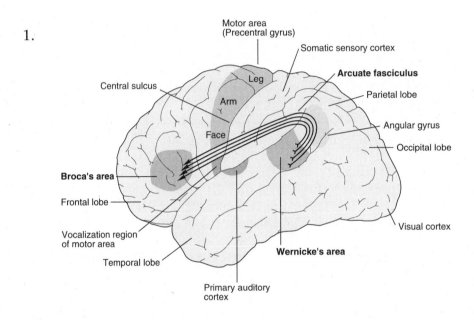

2.

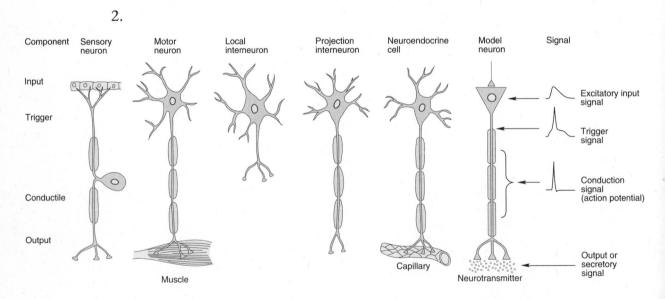

3. See Table 2–1 in the textbook (p. 33) for correct entries.

3 & 4

The Neuron and Neuronal Proteins

Overview

The functional differences between the sensory and motor neurons of the monosynaptic component of the reflex circuit, described in Chapter 2, are the result of cytological (morphological) and molecular differences that arise from different patterns of gene expression in these two types of neurons. To truly understand the function of neurons at the cellular level we must understand these patterns of gene expression.

The direct result of gene expression is the synthesis of proteins. Appropriate proteins must be synthesized in each neuron and targeted to specific cellular compartments (membranes, secretory granules, cytosol, etc.), often to particular locations within a compartment (e.g., to the node of Ranvier membranes or the presynaptic membrane). Proteins are directed to their appropriate compartment by information encoded in their mRNA.

Cytosolic proteins, such as enzymes, are synthesized on free polyribosomes in the cell body. Secretory proteins are synthesized on polyribosomes associated with the rough endoplasmic reticulum, then introduced into the lumen of the endoplasmic reticulum by cotranslational transport, processed there, moved into the Golgi apparatus in transport vesicles, further processed there, and pinched off the Golgi apparatus in secretory vesicles in preparation for release. Membrane-spanning proteins (and other membrane proteins) are synthesized on polyribosomes associated with the rough endoplasmic reticulum, where they are introduced into the membrane of the endoplasmic reticulum by cotranslational transport, processed there, moved into the Golgi apparatus in transport vesicles, further processed there, and pinched off the Golgi apparatus in transport vesicles in preparation for insertion into the appropriate membrane.

The unique morphology of neurons — the functional and structural polarization and the occurrence of long processes (axons and dendrites) — necessitates transport mechanisms to assure that the proteins synthesized in the cell body arrive at their appropriate destinations efficiently. Membrane proteins and secretory proteins are transported quickly down the axon in membrane-bound organelles (secretory vesicles, transport vesicles, etc.) along microtubule tracks, powered by the ATPase kinesin. This mechanism is called anterograde axonal transport. Cytosolic proteins (such as enzymes) and cytoskeletal components move out from the cell body by the slow mechanism of axoplasmic flow. Recycled secretory vesicles and other membrane components, as well as substances such as growth factors, are transported from nerve terminals to the cell body by retrograde axonal transport, a mechanism similar to anterograde axonal transport but powered by the ATPase dynein.

The neuronal cytoskeleton gives neurons their unique shapes, allows them to grow in a directed fashion, and provides tracks for anterograde and retrograde transport. Microtubules, neurofilaments, and microfilaments make up this important neuronal constituent.

Myelin, the electrical insulation medium of the nervous system, is contributed by glial cells: oligodendrocytes in the central nervous system and Schwann cells in the peripheral nervous system. The myelin sheath surrounding axons assures efficient conduction of action potentials.

Objectives

1. Understanding the genetic basis for the similarities and differences among different types of neurons.

2. Understanding the subcellular and cellular specialization of the dorsal root ganglion sensory neurons and spinal motor neurons that constitute the monosynaptic component of the stretch reflex.

3. Understanding the synthesis and fate of the different classes of proteins that neurons express.

4. Understanding the role of specialized transport mechanisms within the neuron.

5. Understanding the basic constituents of the neuronal cytoskeleton and their role in determining neuronal structure, in directing growth, and in axonal transport.

6. Understanding how the myelin sheath around the axon is formed by glial cells in the central and peripheral nervous system and its role in axonal conduction.

■ COMPLETION PROBLEMS

1. Each neuron synthesizes four main types of proteins (macromolecules) that define its characteristic structure and properties: _____, _____, _____, and _____.

2. In spinal motor neurons almost all of the presynaptic boutons are located on the _____; only 5% are located on or close to the _____.

3. In the monosynaptic component of the stretch reflex circuit each motor neuron receives _____ to _____ contacts from a single sensory neuron, and each sensory neuron contacts _____ to _____ motor neurons.

4. In the stretch reflex circuit the transmitter used by motor neurons at neuromuscular junctions is _____; the transmitter presumably used by the sensory neurons at their synapses with the motor neuron is _____.

5. In spinal motor neurons the spike trigger zone is located at the _____ and _____, parts of the axon that are not covered with myelin.

6. In spinal motor neurons the average total length of the 7 to 18 dendrites issuing from the cell body is about _____ cell body diameters; the mean path length for all motor neurons is _____ mm.

7. In a spinal motor neuron synaptic boutons cover about _____ of the surface area of the axon hillock and cell body and _____ of the dendritic membrane.

8. The myelin that ensheaths axons in the central nervous system is formed by _____, while in the peripheral nervous system the myelin is formed by _____.

9. The interruptions in the myelin sheath along an axon are called _____.

10. Myelin-associated glycoprotein (MAG) is thought to be an _____ involved in the initiation of the myelination process in peripheral axons.

11. Antibodies generated in response to myelin basic proteins injected into a mammal cause _____, which is an experimental model for demyelinating diseases like multiple sclerosis.

12. The nucleolus contains the specific portion of the DNA that encodes the RNA of future _____.

13. Like other cells, neurons make three classes of proteins: (1) protein synthesized in the _____; (2) proteins synthesized in the _____ that are later imported into the nucleus or mitochondria; and (3) proteins synthesized in association with the membranes of the _____.

14. There are three distinct membrane systems in a cell (e.g., a neuron): the major membrane system, _____, and _____.

15. The major membrane system consists of (1) _____, (2) _____, (3) _____, (4) _____, (5) _____, and (6) _____.

16. The three categories of proteins associated with the cell's membrane system are: (1) proteins that remain attached to the membranes of the _____; (2) proteins that remain in the _____ of the endoplasmic reticulum or _____ sacs; and (3) proteins distributed in _____ vesicles or organelles such as _____.

17. Membrane proteins are of three subtypes: _____, _____ and _____.

18. Membrane proteins, luminal proteins, and secretory proteins are syn-

thesized on polyribosomes that become associated with the membranes of the _____.

19. Proteins synthesized on polyribosomes associated with the endoplasmic reticulum (membrane and secretory proteins) are incorporated into membrane or transferred to the endoplasmic reticulum's lumen by _____, while nuclear and mitochondrial proteins are incorporated into these structures after synthesis on cytosolic polyribosomes by _____.

20. Membrane components leave the Golgi apparatus in a variety of _____; in the neuron _____ or _____ are particularly important.

21. The cytoskeleton gives a neuron its characteristic shape, and provides the tracks for fast axonal transport. Three types of filamentous proteins that contribute to the cytoskeleton are _____, _____, and _____.

22. Newly synthesized membrane and secretory proteins after processing in the Golgi apparatus are moved in vesicles by _____ away from their sites of synthesis in the cell body, along tracks of _____, by the ATPase motor molecule _____.

23. Recycled membrane constituents and molecules such as growth factors from nerve terminals are moved to the cell body by _____, along tracks of _____ by the ATPase motor molecule _____.

24. Of the two kinetic components of slow axoplasmic flow, the fastest component moves _____ and small amounts of a large number of _____ proteins, while the slower moves predominantly (75%) _____ and _____ subunits.

25. Microfilaments are made up of two polarized polymer strands of _____ wound into a helix.

26. Microtubules are polarized alternating heteropolymers of _____ and _____, subunits that can each bind two molecules of _____, one of which is hydrolysable to _____.

27. A microtubule is made up of _____ protofilaments and has a diameter of _____ nm, while its longest length in an axon is _____.

28. Each actin monomer of a microfilament can bind a molecule of _____ that can be hydrolyzed to _____.

29. Neurofilaments have a diameter of _____ nm, while micro-filaments have a diameter of _____ nm.

30. The hydrolyzation state of bound nucleotide phosphate determines the _____ and _____ dynamics of microtubules and microfilaments.

■ *TRUE/FALSE QUESTIONS*
(If false, explain why)

1. Less than one-tenth of a spinal motor neuron's total volume is in the cell body. _____

2. A muscle spindle is a receptor that is sensitive to stretch. _____

3. In spinal motor neurons most excitatory synapses are close to the cell body, while inhibitory ones are further out along the dendrites. _____

4. In a spinal motor neuron the change in membrane potential resulting from synaptic input is monitored at the trigger zone, where the cell membrane is rich in acetylcholine receptors. _____

5. A specific transporter protein for choline is expressed by sensory neurons but not by motor neurons. _____

6. Spines are specialized postsynaptic structures on the dendrites of many central neurons, and the molecular machinery for protein synthesis is frequently situated just beneath these structures. _____

7. Recurrent collaterals are the sites in spinal motor neurons at which synaptic inputs are integrated and the decision to fire an action potential is made. _____

8. Myelin has a similar composition to plasma membrane, being 30% lipid and 70% protein. _____

9. The distance between nodes of Ranvier on a sensory axon from a muscle spindle is 1 to 1.5 mm. _____

10. Demyelination of the type seen in diseases like multiple sclerosis or *shiverer* mice causes a decrease in axonal conduction speed, but remarkably gives rise to no overt behavioral symptoms. _____

11. The nucleolus is particularly prominent in secretory cells like neurons. _____

12. All the DNA necessary to encode all the proteins of the cell and its various organelles is found in the nucleus. _____

13. The cytosol is a gel consisting of water-soluble proteins and a variety of insoluble filaments that form the cytoskeleton. _____

14. Certain proteins are expressed by all neurons in general, while other are specific to particular neuronal types. _____

15. With the exception of a few proteins encoded by the mitochondrial genome, essentially all the proteins of a neuron are made in the cell body from mRNA originating in the nucleus. _____

16. The information that determines whether a protein will be synthesized on the rough endoplasmic reticulum, and thus will become associated with the membrane systems of the cell, is encoded in the mRNA for that protein. _____

17. The mRNAs that encode cytosolic and imported (nucleus and mitochondria) proteins are translated on free cytosolic polyribosomes. _____

18. Membrane and secretory proteins are extensively modified after synthesis as they travel through the endoplasmic reticulum and Golgi apparatus into transport vesicles. _____

19. Cytosolic enzymes are transported to the nerve terminal by anterograde axonal transport. _____

20. Toxins like colchicine and vinblastin that disrupt actin filaments interfere with fast axonal transport. _____

21. Materials packaged in large membrane-bound organelles (transport vesicles) that are part of the lysosomal system are moved back to the cell body by retrograde axonal transport for recycling. _____

22. Slow axoplasmic flow is both anterograde and retrograde. _____

23. Slow axoplasmic flow transports proteins packaged in membrane-bound organelles. _____

24. Neurofilaments are complex polymers consisting of coiled-coils of cytokeratin proteins that rarely, if ever, depolymerize. _____

25. Neurofilaments are particularly important in controlling cell movements such as growth and elongation of axons and dendrites. _____

SYNTHETIC QUESTIONS AND QUANTITATIVE PROBLEMS

1. Identify the organelles responsible for the synthesis and processing of neuronal proteins.

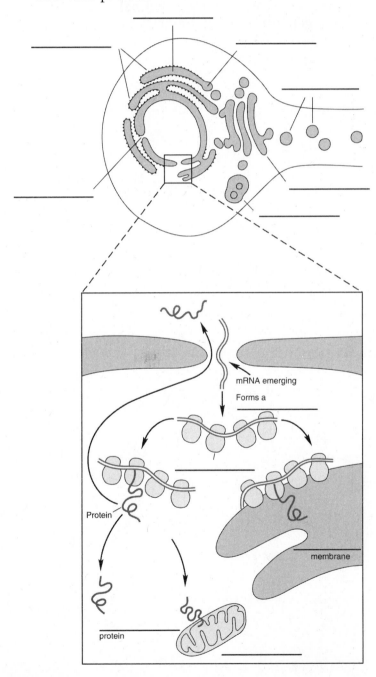

mRNA emerging

Forms a ___

Protein

___ membrane

protein

Figure 3–1

2. Trace the synthesis and fate of a second neuroactive peptide and an enzyme involved in the synthesis of a small-molecule transmitter (e.g., choline acetyltransferase that synthesizes acetylcholine from acetyl-coenzyme A and choline) from the site production of mRNA in the nucleus to the site of transmitter/peptide release at a distance presynaptic nerve terminal. How do neuroactive peptides get into secretory vesicles for release at nerve terminals? How do small-molecule transmitters get into synaptic vesicles for release at nerve terminals?

ANSWERS

◼ COMPLETION PROBLEMS

1. enzymes; structural proteins; membrane constituents; secretory products

2. dendritic branches; cell body

3. 2; 6; 500; 1,000

4. acetylcholine; (L-)glutamate

5. axon hillock; initial segment

6. 20; 1.5

7. 1/2; 3/4

8. oligodendrocytes; Schwann cells

9. nodes of Ranvier

10. adhesion molecule

11. experimental allergic encephalomyelitis

12. ribosomes

13. cytoplasm; cytoplasm; endoplasmic reticulum

14. lysosomes; mitochondria

15. the nuclear envelope; endoplasmic reticulum; Golgi apparatus; secretory granules; endosomes; plasma membrane

16. endoplasmic reticulum; lumen; Golgi; secretory; lysosomes

17. membrane-spanning; anchored; associated

18. rough endoplasmic reticulum

19. cotranslational transport; posttranslational importation

20. vesicles; secretory vesicles; synaptic vesicles

21. microtubules; neurofilaments; microfilaments

22. fast anterograde axonal transport; microtubules; kinesin

23. fast retrograde axonal transport; microtubules; dynein

24. actin; cytosolic; microtubules; neurofilaments

25. actin

26. α-tubulin; β-tubulin; GTP; GDP

27. 13; 25; 0.1

28. ATP; ADP

29. 10; 7

30. polymerization; depolymerization

■ TRUE/FALSE QUESTIONS

1. True

2. True

3. False. In spinal motor neurons most inhibitory synapses are close to the cell body, while excitatory ones are further out along the dendrites.

4. False. In a spinal motor neuron the change in membrane potential resulting from synaptic input is monitored at the trigger zone, where the cell membrane is rich in *voltage-gated sodium channels.*

5. False. A specific transporter protein for choline is expressed by motor neurons but not by sensory neurons.

6. True

7. False. The *trigger zone* (axon hillock and initial segment) is the site in spinal motor neurons at which synaptic inputs are integrated and the decision to fire an action potential is made.

8. False. Myelin has a similar composition to plasma membrane, being 70% lipid and 30% protein.

9. True

10. False. Demyelination of the type seen in diseases like multiple sclerosis or in genetic defects like shiverer in mice causes a decrease in axonal conduction speed and give rise to several behavioral symptoms.

11. True

12. False. *Almost* all the DNA necessary to encode the proteins of the cell and its various organelles is found in the nucleus; some is found in the mitochondria.

13. True

14. True

15. True

16. True

17. True

18. True

19. False. Cytosolic enzymes are transported to the nerve terminal by *slow axonal flow.*

20. False. Toxins like colchicine and vinblastin that disrupt *microtubules* interfere with fast axonal transport.

21. True

22. False. Slow axoplasmic flow is anterograde only.

23. False. Slow axoplasmic flow transports unpackaged soluble proteins and cytoskeletal elements.

24. True

25. False. *Micro*filaments are particularly important in controlling cell movements such as growth and elongation of axons and dendrites.

■ SYNTHETIC QUESTIONS AND QUANTITATIVE PROBLEMS

1. See Figure 4–2 in the textbook, p. 59.

2. The mRNA for the enzyme would pass through a nuclear pore into the cytoplasm of the cell body, where the enzyme would be synthesized on free cytosolic polyribosomes. The finished enzyme would move to the presynaptic terminals in the fast component of slow axoplasmic flow. In the presynaptic terminals, this enzyme would synthesize the small-molecule transmitter and the transmitter would be loaded into synaptic vesicles for release by transporters in the vesicle membrane. The vesicles could be released, recycled, refilled; and rereleased several times in the terminals without any necessity for return to the cell body.

   The mRNA for the neuroactive peptide would pass through a nuclear pore into the cytoplasm of the cell body, where the mRNA would interact polyribosomes that become associated with the rough endoplasmic reticulum. On the rough endoplasmic reticulum the peptide precursor protein would be synthesized and introduced into the lumen of the endoplasmic reticulum by cotranslational transport. Once in the lumen of the endoplasmic reticulum, the precursor protein would be processed into the neuroactive peptide in stages, beginning in the endoplasmic reticulum but continuing as the protein moved from the endoplasmic reticulum into the Golgi apparatus in transport vesicles. The finished (or nearly finished) neuroactive peptide would emerge from the Golgi apparatus in a secretory granule (vesicle) that would move to the nerve terminal for release by fast anterograde axonal transport. After release, the secretory granule would be recycled from the presynaptic membrane and transported back to the cell body by fast retrograde axonal transport, where it would merge with the Golgi apparatus and be refilled.

   Thus, we can see that small-molecule transmitters and secreted neuroactive peptides differ fundamentally in their preparation for release; neuroactive peptides are loaded into secretory granules (vesicles) for release only in the cell body, whereas small-molecule transmitters are loaded into vesicles for release at the release sites in the nerve terminal.

5

The Nervous System

Overview

The functional and structural aspects of the nervous system are inseparable. Only by understanding the functional anatomy of the nervous system can the cellular analysis, which we are about to embark upon in upcoming chapters, be placed in its proper functional and behavioral perspective.

The nervous system can be divided into the central nervous system (CNS), made up of the brain and spinal cord, and the peripheral nervous system (PNS) made up of sensory and autonomic ganglia and peripheral nerves. The somatic branch of the PNS sends somatic and special sensory information into the CNS and sends out motor commands to somatic muscles that are generated in the CNS. The autonomic branch of the PNS controls the viscera and sends visceral sensory information to the CNS.

Even the simplest behaviors involve the integrated activity of several distinct sensory, motor, and motivational pathways in the CNS. Each pathway contains relay nuclei and each of these nuclei has several functional subdivisions that process and relay information onto the next stage in the pathway. Two or more parallel pathways may process similar or diverse information and converge at "higher" centers. Diverse sensory and motor pathways converge in association areas in the cerebral cortex, areas that control our most complex behaviors and cognitive functions.

Within a sensory or motor pathway neurons are usually arranged in precise topographic fashion, so that the arrangement of sensory space or motor output in the body is represented consistently throughout the CNS.

Most pathways within the CNS cross (decussate), so that the left body side is controlled by and represented in the right side of the brain and vice versa. These basic principles of organization within the CNS can be seen at all levels, from the spinal cord through the brain stem to the highest levels of the cerebral cortex.

Objectives

1. Understanding the functional anatomy of the human central and peripheral nervous systems.

2. Understanding how new imaging techniques help us explore the functional anatomy of the human central nervous system.

3. Understanding the major perceptual, movement, and motivational systems of the central nervous system.

4. Understanding the topographic arrangement of sensory and motor representations in the central nervous system and the functional implications of this organization.

■ *COMPLETION PROBLEMS*

1. _____ (PET) provides images of live, real-time brain functioning.

2. The term "tomography" implies that an image is restricted to a single _____ or _____ of tissue.

3. Like conventional radiography, _____ (CAT) produces X-ray images of structure, but also reveals subtle differences in tissues that cannot be detected in conventional X-ray images.

4. PET scans can identify areas where _____ is actively being metabolized. For this purpose the non-metabolizable molecule

_____ is introduced into the cerebral blood stream and detected with a positron-emitting isotope that binds tightly to molecules of _____, which are trapped intracellularly in actively metabolizing neurons.

5. _____ (MRI) can reveal detailed images that enable clinicians to locate lesions of the brain noninvasively.

6. The peripheral nervous system has _____ and _____ divisions.

7. The peripheral nervous system consists of the peripheral _____ and _____.

8. The autonomic motor system consists of the antagonistic _____ and _____ systems and the _____ nervous system that controls the smooth muscle of the gut.

9. The peripheral axons of somatic _____ are often considered part of the somatic division of the peripheral nervous system, despite the fact that the cell bodies are located in the spinal cord.

10. The sensory neurons that constitute the somatic division of the peripheral nervous system have their cell bodies in the _____ and _____ ganglia.

11. The central nervous system consists of seven major regions: (1) the _____; (2) _____; (3) _____; (4) _____; (5) _____; (6) _____;and (7) _____.

12. _____ roots carry sensory information into the spinal cord, while _____ roots carry outgoing motor axons that innervate somatic muscles as well as axons of the _____ and _____ systems.

13. There are _____ pairs of spinal nerves and _____ pairs of cranial nerves.

14. The surface convolutions of the cerebral cortex consist of groves called _____ that separate elevated regions called _____.

15. The thalamus and hypothalamus together form the _____.

16. The term _____ indicates the direction toward the head.

17. The _____ cortex occupies the medial wall of the lateral sulcus, also known as the _____ fissure.

18. The _____ lobe, although not really a distinct cerebral cortical lobe, is a continuous band of cortex that is considered a unit because it forms neural circuits that play an important role in learning, memory, and emotions.

19. _____ motor and sensory cortex is directly involved with lower-level processing of sensory information or motor commands, while _____ cortex integrates diverse information for purposeful action.

20. Three deep-lying structures are part of the cerebral hemispheres: the _____, _____ and _____.

21. The _____ is the main modulator of the autonomic motor system.

22. The _____, which is part of the limbic system, plays a particularly important role in memory, while the _____, also part of the limbic system, plays an important role in controlling emotions.

23. Sensory, motor, and motivational systems are interconnected within and among themselves through _____ nuclei, and these nuclei consist of _____ interneurons that mediate inhibitory and excitatory effects within the nucleus and _____ interneurons that transmit the output of the nucleus.

24. Almost all sensory information that reaches the cerebral cortex is first processed in the _____.

25. The _____ and _____, two of the seven major regions of the brain, are thought to be primarily involved in the planning, timing, and patterning of movement, and in motor learning.

26. The _____ organization of sensory and motor pathways creates _____ of sensory space and motor effectors in functionally discrete brain areas.

27. The major sensory, motor, and motivational systems of the brain each have several anatomically and functionally _____ that perform specialized tasks in parallel.

28. Most major and sensory pathways within the central nervous system cross (or _____).

29. Central nervous structures that contain only crossing axons are called
_____.

30. The _____ contains crossing axons that interconnect the two cerebral hemispheres.

■ SYNTHETIC QUESTIONS AND QUANTITATIVE PROBLEMS

1. Identify the subdivisions of the embryonic and mature central nervous system.

Three-Vesicle Stage	Five-Vesicle Stage	Mature Structures Derived from Vesicle	Related Cavity	
1. _____	1a. Telencephalon (endbrain)	1. _____	_____	ventricles
	1b. Diencephalon	2. _____	_____	ventricle
2. _____	2. Mesencephalon (midbrain)	3. _____	Cerebral _____	
3. _____	3a. Metencephalon (afterbrain)	4. _____	_____	ventricle
	3b. Myelencephalon (medullary brain)	6. _____	_____	ventricle
4. Caudal part of neural tube	4. _____	7. _____	Central _____	

2. Identify the structures indicated on this midsaggital human brain section.

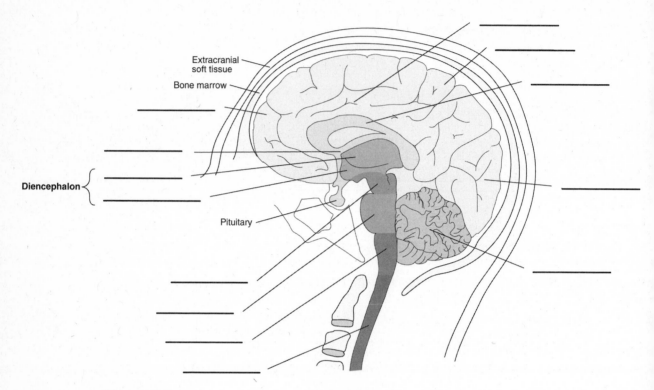

Figure 5–1

3. Enter the missing labels on these schematic drawings of a human brain.

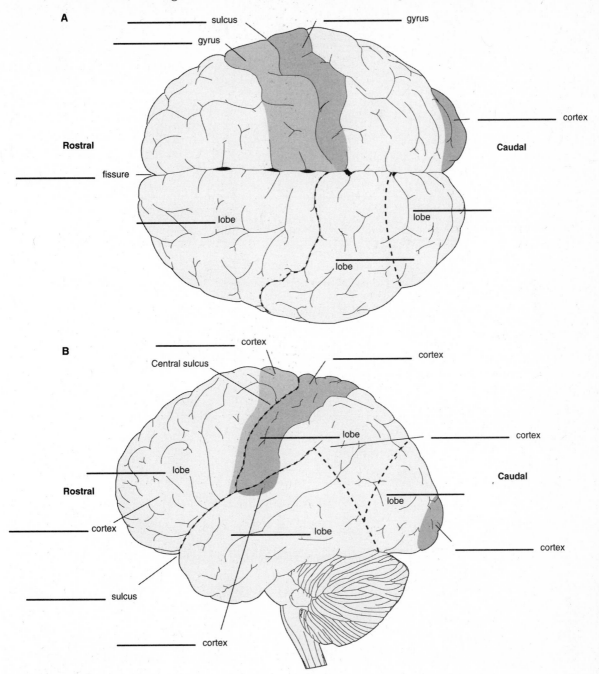

Figure 5–2

4. Trace the transcerebral pathway of sensory information leading from mechanical stimulation of the skin on a finger to the coordinated movement of the finger in response to the stimulus.

5. If the human optic chiasm is cut, what parts of the visual field would be lost?

ANSWERS

■ COMPLETION PROBLEMS

1. position emission tomography

2. plane; section

3. computer assisted tomography

4. glucose; 2-deoxyglucose; deoxyglucose 6-phosphate

5. magnetic resonance imaging

6. somatic; autonomic

7. ganglia; peripheral nerves

8. sympathetic; parasympathetic; enteric

9. motor neurons

10. cranial; dorsal root

11. spinal cord; medulla; pons; cerebellum; midbrain; diencephalon; cerebral hemispheres

12. dorsal; ventral; sympathetic; parasympathetic

13. 31; 12

14. sulci; gyri

15. diencephalon

16. rostral

17. insular; Sylvian

18. limbic

19. primary; association

20. basal ganglia; hippocampus; amygdala

21. hypothalamus

22. hippocampus; amygdala

23. relay; local; projection

24. thalamus

25. pons; cerebellum

26. topographical; neural maps

27. distinct subsystems

28. decussate

29. commissures

30. corpus callosum

SYNTHETIC QUESTIONS AND QUANTITATIVE PROBLEMS

1. See Table 5–1 in the textbook, p. 77.

2. See Figure 5–6B in the textbook, p. 80.

3. See Figure 5–8 in the textbook, p. 82.

4. The pathway is as follows (see Figure 5–9 in the textbook, p. 85). A primary mechanosensory afferent from the skin (cell body in a dorsal root ganglion) ascends in the spinal cord to a dorsal column relay nucleus, the axons of which ascend (decussating in the brain stem) to a thalamic relay nucleus. Axons from these relay neurons ascend to the primary somatic sensory cortex (postcentral gyrus), whose neurons project to the primary motor cortex (precental gyrus). These motor neurons project to the spinal cord (as well as other, parallel subcortical motor centers). The spinal cord neural circuitry forms the final efferent pathway to skeletal motor neurons.

5. In the largely overlapping visual fields of the two eyes in humans, the left visual field is surveyed by the right temporal (closest to the temple) hemiretina and the right visual field is surveyed by the left temporal hemiretina, while the left visual field is surveyed by the left nasal (closest to the nose) hemiretina of the left eye and the right visual field is surveyed by the right nasal hemiretina of the right eye. If the optic chiasm is cut in a human, the perceived visual field would remain largely intact (some of the peripheral visual field on both sides would be lost), because both the right and left visual fields would be represented in the left and right primary visual cortex by the nondecussating axons from the temporal hemiretina of each eye. There would be no binocular representation in either visual cortex, however, because the decussating axons from the nasal would be severed.

6

Development of the Nervous System

Overview

In his autobiography published in 1917 Santiago y Ramón y Cajal crystal-lized the important findings and questions that confront modern develop-mental neuroscientists with the following colorful passage: "I noticed that every ramification, dendritic or axonic, in the course of formation, passes through a chaotic period, so to speak, a period of trials, during which there are sent out at random experimental conductors most of which are des-tined to disappear . . . . What mysterious forces precede the appearance of processes, promote their growth and ramification, . . . and finally establish those protoplasmic kisses, the intercellular articulations, which seem to constitute the final ecstasy of an epic love story."

The establishment of the mature pattern of synaptic connections in the vertebrate nervous system occurs in six major stages:

(1) Signals from the mesoderm in the early embryo induce ectodermal cells to form a uniform population of precursor cells.
(2) The precursor cells begin to divide and diversify giving rise to glial cells and immature neurons.
(3) Immature neurons migrate from their germinal zone to their final positions.
(4) Neurons extend and project axons into the vicinity of their eventual targets.
(5) The neurons form synaptic connections with selected target cells.
(6) The initial pattern of synaptic connections is pruned by competition among neurons for trophic factors and by physiological activity to form the mature pattern of connections.

An important aspect of the earlier steps of this program is the genetic commitment to a particular fate and the differentiation that realizes that fate. Commitment can be viewed as a relatively irreversible step to a particular program of gene expression, and differentiation as the readout of that program. These processes are set into motion by signals that alter gene expression by interacting with transcriptional regulatory proteins within the cells. The signals may be inherited from ancestor cells or provided by neighboring cells, i.e., the genes are regulated by cell lineage or cell-cell interactions. The signals that arise through cell lineage (intrinsic signals) can result by unequal partitioning of molecules between daughter cells during a division. Signals arising through cell-cell interactions (extrinsic signals) can be presented on the surface of neighboring cells or may be diffusible molecules released at some distance. Cell-cell interaction plays a primary role in the development of the vertebrate nervous system. Commitment and differentiation can occur in steps. Thus, a precursor cell gives rise to progeny that are committed to a neuronal fate but not yet committed to a particular transmitter type; commitment to transmitter type occurs on further interaction with the developmental environment.

The migration of neurons and the guidance of axons to their targets are mediated by chemical cues that may be present in the extracellular matrix on the surface of neurons or glial cells, or may be released into the vicinity of the migrating neuron or outgrowing axons. These cues may be attractive or repulsive. The establishment of initial synaptic contacts between a neuron and its appropriate target is thought to be mediated by direct cell-cell interaction between neuron and target. The job of axonal outgrowth, the reading of guidance cues, and the initial formation of synapses are all accomplished by the growth cone, the remarkable dynamic structure at the tip of the growing axon. The initial formation of synaptic connections may involve a precise matching of presynaptic surface molecules and postsynaptic surface recognition molecules (the chemoaffinity hypothesis).

During development the interaction between a neuron and its postsynaptic target is dynamic and cooperative. Molecules released at the surface of the axon terminal orchestrate the synthesis, turnover, distribution, and properties of postsynaptic receptors; trophic molecules released or presented by the target promote neuronal survival and synapse stabilization. Electrical activity in target cells also influences receptor distribution and possibly synapse stabilization. The initial pattern of synaptic connections between a population of neurons and their targets is often restricted by competition for trophic factors from the target, and the presynaptic cells that lose out in this competition die in a process known as programmed cell death.

Thus, in the nervous system of vertebrates during development there is an overproduction of neurons and an exuberant formation of synaptic connections, both of which are pruned back to produce the functional pattern of connections seen in the mature nervous system. As we shall see in future chapters, experience (sensory or motor) can influence these pruning processes to assure that the final pattern of connections adapts to environmental requirements.

Objectives

1. Understanding the intrinsic factors (from cell lineage) and extrinsic factors (from neighboring cells) that influence the pattern of gene expression in developing neuronal precursors.

2. Understanding the importance of neuronal migration, axonal pathfinding, and cell-cell interaction in establishing appropriate synaptic connections.

3. Understanding the importance of neuronal competition for trophic factors provided by target tissues, pruning, and programmed cell death in the formation of the mature pattern of synaptic connections.

■ *TRUE/FALSE QUESTIONS*
(If false, explain why)

1. Even in the nematode *Caenorhabditis elegans,* whose cell lineage during development is invariant, signals from other cells can have a role in determining the fate of neurons. _____

2. Cell-cell interactions play a critical role in the differentiation of most types of neurons in the vertebrate nervous system. _____

3. Both diffusible molecules and nondiffusible cell-surface molecules can mediate signals between cells during development that determine cell fate. _____

4. The intracellular signaling mechanisms involved in neural development in invertebrates are not similar to those observed in vertebrates. _____

5. In vertebrate embryos ectodermal cells that do not acquire neural properties give rise to skin. _____

6. In vertebrate embryos the differentiation of the neural plate from uncommitted ectoderm is induced by cells in the adjacent endoderm. _____

7. Some of the genes that differentiate cells in the fly and human nervous systems are conserved in structure and function. _____

8. In higher vertebrates the segmentation of the hindbrain and perhaps also the midbrain and forebrain is thought to result from cell interactions with the adjacent developing somites. _____

9. Neurons and neuroblasts do not migrate after they have extended axons. _____

10. All the different neurons that eventually populate the several layers of the cerebral cortex derive from neuroblasts that originate in the ventricular proliferation zone. _____

11. In the technique of [³H]thymidine birthdating, heavily labeled cells are those that were born just prior to the [³H]thymidine pulse. _____

12. [³H]thymidine birthdating shows that neurons born at a late stage of cerebral cortical development end up in the deepest cortical layers, while those born at earlier times end up in progressively more superficial layers. _____

13. In the cerebral cortex neurons born at later times must migrate past those that have already achieved their final position in the cortex. _____

14. The inverted cortical development seen in the mutant *reeler* mouse indicates that a neuron's birth date and developmental history are more important in determining its morphology, properties, and connections than is its final position in the cortex. _____

15. The fate of cortical cells is determined more by migratory route, while the fate of neural crest cells is determined more by birth date. _____

16. The establishment of appropriate retinotectal connections during

development in amphibians is a good example of early and specific axonal pathfinding. _____

17. Sperry's studies of inverted eye regeneration in newts show that regenerating axons make new, behaviorally appropriate connections rather than reconnecting to their original postsynaptic targets. _____

18. During development in vertebrates, outgrowing axons of motor neurons segregate themselves into different spinal roots so that they may reach their appropriate muscle targets. _____

19. During development in vertebrates, outgrowing axons of motor neurons recognize specific cues within the limb plexus that guide them to their appropriate muscle targets. _____

20. During development in vertebrates, outgrowing axons of motor neurons will not segregate into their appropriate motor nerves if the target muscles are ablated. _____

21. Integrins mediate interaction between the cell surface of growth cones and extracellular matrix molecules like laminin and fibronectin. _____

22. Diffusible chemical factors released by target tissues can attract outgrowing cones to these tissues in a process known as chemotropism. _____

23. In amphibians axons from the retina may be guided to their appropriate place in the tectum by molecules that repel growth cones. _____

24. In vertebrate development, when a muscle fiber is first innervated by a motor neuron, the density of receptors at both the synaptic and extrasynaptic sites increases. _____

25. The density of synaptic receptors in mature vertebrate muscle is only 10 times the density at extrasynaptic sites. _____

26. The disappearance of extrasynaptic acetylcholine receptors during development of the vertebrate neuromuscular junction is controlled by a chemotrophic mechanism. _____

27. Acetylcholine receptors at the vertebrate neuromuscular junction have a shorter half-life than those at extrasynaptic sites on the same muscle fiber. _____

28. Elimination of synapses through neuronal competition is a regular part of the development of the vertebrate neuromuscular junction. _____

29. Experimentally induced changes in the size of a neuronal target during development affect the survival of postmitotic (fully differentiated) neurons, but do not affect the population of neuronal precursors. _____

30. Vertebrates and invertebrates may possess common molecular mechanisms for programmed cell death. _____

31. Survival of spinal motor neurons during development of the mouse requires nerve growth factor. _____

32. Death of neurons is commonplace in normal development of the vertebrate embryo, often resulting in the loss of up to half of all the neurons initially generated. _____

■ COMPLETION PROBLEMS

1. The signals that determine the program of gene expression that leads to neuronal differentiation may be intrinsic (from _____) or extrinsic (from _____). Intrinsic signals can result by unequal _____ of molecules between daughter cells during a division, while extrinsic signals can be presented on the _____ of neighboring cells or may be _____ molecules released at some distance.

2. The entire vertebrate nervous system develops from the _____, the _____ layer of the early embryo.

3. In vertebrate embryos the neural plate first appears as a thickened _____.

4. The segmental form of the developing hindbrain in higher vertebrates can easily be observed in conspicuous dorsal swellings termed _____, which may be responsible for the organization of individual _____ nuclei.

5. In vertebrate embryos, after induction by signals from the organizer region, cells within the neural plate differentiate into _____ or _____.

6. The neural crest is a _____ and _____ group of cells that emerges from the _____ region of the neural tube.

7. Neural crest cells migrate to different peripheral locations, where they form the _____ and _____ cells of the _____ and _____ nervous systems (ganglia), the _____ cells of the adrenal medulla, the _____ of the skin, enteric neurons, and the _____ tissues of the face and skull.

8. The sympathoadrenal sublineages of the neural crest comprise the major _____ descendants of the neural crest: sympathetic neurons adrenal _____ cells and _____ of the sympathetic ganglia.

9. During development of the vertebrate central nervous system the eventual position of many different classes of neurons is achieved by the _____ of neuroblasts from the site of their _____ in the ventricular zone of the neuroepithelium.

10. The term _____ indicates the time at which a dividing precursor undergoes its final round of cell division to become a _____ neuron.

11. Transplant studies of the cerebral cortex show that the cortical layer for which a cell is destined is determined just before the cell is _____; thus _____ occurs prior to migration.

12. In the cerebral cortex _____ glial cells that span the _____ guide the migration of neurons from the _____ to their final destinations.

13. The neuronal growth cone is a specialized _____ and _____ apparatus containing finger-like projections called _____, which extend and guide growing axons to their targets.

14. The new membrane added at the growth cone to extend an axon is synthesized in the _____, packaged into _____, and transported along _____ that extend into the growth cone.

15. According to the _____ hypothesis, individual neurons

acquire distinctive molecular markers, or _____ molecules, early in development, and the establishment of appropriate connections between neurons would depend on the correct _____ of molecules on the _____ of pre- and postsynaptic neurons.

16. Three classes of glycoproteins act as cell adhesion molecules that help guide axonal outgrowth: molecules of the _____ superfamily, _____, and _____.

17. Development of the vertebrate neuromuscular junction involves changes in the _____ and _____ of acetylcholine receptors, changes in the _____ of the receptors, and an increase in the _____ of nerve muscle contacts.

18. The distribution of acetylcholine receptors in a vertebrate muscle fiber is changed following innervation during development by _____ of preexisting receptors in the membrane and _____ of receptors at the synaptic site, and by insertion of _____ receptors at or near the synaptic site.

19. Acetylcholine receptors in embryonic rat muscle have a relatively _____ conductance and a _____ open time when acetylcholine is bound, while in mature rat muscle these receptors have a relatively _____ conductance and a _____ open time when acetylcholine is bound.

20. The competition among neurons at the developing vertebrate neuromuscular junction appears to involve access to _____ provided by the muscles.

21. The process of overproduction of neurons followed by drastic reduction in their numbers is known as _____.

■ SYNTHETIC QUESTIONS AND QUANTITATIVE PROBLEMS

1. Give an example from the development of the nervous system in invertebrates where differentiation of neurons is controlled by cell lineage and where differentiation of neurons is controlled by cell-cell interaction.

ANSWERS

TRUE/FALSE QUESTIONS

1. True

2. True

3. True

4. False. The intracellular signaling mechanisms involved in neural development in invertebrates are *similar* to those observed in vertebrates.

5. True

6. False. In vertebrate embryos the differentiation of the neural plate from uncommitted ectoderm is induced by cells in the adjacent *meso*derm.

7. True

8. False. In higher vertebrates the segmentation of the hindbrain and perhaps also the midbrain and forebrain is thought to result from cell interactions that are *intrinsic to the neural tube*.

9. False. Some neurons and neuroblasts do migrate after they have extended axons.

10. True

11. False. In the technique of [^{3}H]thymidine birthdating, heavily labeled cells are those that had been born a short time *after* the [^{3}H]thymidine pulse.

12. False. [^{3}H]thymidine birthdating shows that neurons born at an *early* stage of cerebral cortical development end up in the deepest cortical

layers, while those born at *later* times end up in progressively more superficial layers.

13. True

14. True

15. False. The fate of neural crest cells is determined more by migratory route, while the fate of cortical cells is determined more by birthdate.

16. True

17. False. Sperry's studies of inverted eye regeneration in newts show that regenerating axons reconnect to their original postsynaptic targets, rather than making behaviorally appropriate connections.

18. False. During development in vertebrates outgrowing axons of motor neurons are *intermingled in the spinal roots,* but when they reach the base of the developing limb, they segregate themselves into different motor nerve branches so that they may reach their appropriate muscle targets.

19. True

20. False. During development in vertebrates outgrowing axons of motor neurons will segregate into their appropriate motor nerves *even if* the target muscles are ablated.

21. True

22. True

23. True

24. False. In vertebrate development, when a muscle fiber is first innervated by a motor neuron, the density of receptors at the synaptic sites increases, while at extrasynaptic sites it decreases.

25. False. The density of synaptic receptors in mature vertebrate muscle is *several thousandfold greater* than at extrasynaptic sites.

26. False. The disappearance of extrasynaptic acetylcholine receptors during development of the vertebrate neuromuscular junction is controlled by an *electrical* mechanism.

27. False. Acetylcholine receptors at the vertebrate neuromuscular junc-

tion have a much *longer* half-life than those at extrasynaptic sites on the same muscle fiber.

28. True

29. True

30. True

31. False. Survival of spinal motor neurons during development of the mouse does *not* require nerve growth factor.

32. True

■ COMPLETION PROBLEMS

1. cell lineage; cell-cell interaction; partitioning; surface; diffusible

2. ectoderm; outer

3. columnar epithelium

4. rhombomeres; cranial motor nerve

5. neurons; glial cells

6. transient; migratory; dorsal

7. neurons; Schwann; sensory; autonomic; chromaffin; melanocytes; mesenchymal

8. catacholaminergic; chromaffin; SIF

9. migration; proliferation

10. birthday; postmitotic

11. born; commitment

12. radial; neuroepithelium; ventricular zone

13. sensory; motor; filopodia

14. cell body; vesicles; microtubules

15. chemoaffinity; recognition; matcning; surfaces

16. immunoglobulin; cadherins; integrins

17. distribution; stability; functional properties; number

18. redistribution; immobilization; newly synthesized

19. small; long; large; short

20. trophic factors

21. programmed neuronal death

■ SYNTHETIC QUESTIONS AND QUANTITATIVE PROBLEMS

1. In the nematode *Caenorhabditis elegans* specific classes of neurons derive from an invariant pattern of cell divisions that is repeated by series of precursor cells along the body axis. For example, the lineage that gives rise to motor neurons is illustrated in Figure 6–1 of the textbook, p. 92.

   In the fruit fly *Drosophila melanogaster* photoreceptor R7 in each ommatidium of the compound eye differentiates when a precursor cell interacts with a surface molecule present on photoreceptor R8, the first photoreceptor to differentiate in an ommatidium. The gene *sevenless* is thought to encode the receptor on precursor cells for the signal molecule presented by the R8 photoreceptor, which in turn is encoded by the *boss* gene. (See Figure 6–3 in the textbook, p. 94).

7

Ion Channels

Overview

An ion channel is a membrane-spanning protein that creates an aqueous pore in the cell membrane through which ions move in response to the electrochemical driving force acting on them. Different types of channels are selective for specific ion species. Some channels are always open (nongated) or are opened (gated) by electrical, mechanical, or chemical signals. The gating process involves the transfer of energy to the channel by either the electrical field across the membrane, a binding ligand, or mechanical deformation that causes a conformational change in the channel proteins. The activity of ion channels can be antagonized or enhanced by various drugs and toxins that competitively bind to the same sites as an activating ligand or noncompetitively bind to other sites that alter channel gating.

Three gene families encode most of the currently described ion channels. The different channel species within each family are isoforms — with different functions — formed by processes such as alternative RNA splicing. Channel isoforms are expressed at different developmental stages and in different cells and subcellar regions, making possible the design of drugs that act only in particular anatomical or cellular regions in the nervous system.

Objectives

1. Understanding the relation between channel structure and function.

2. Understanding the selectivity of channels.

3. Understanding the types and mechanisms of channel gating.

4. Understanding how drugs and toxins interact with ion channels by competitive and noncompetitive interactions.

5. Understanding channel structural diversity and its relation to channel function.

6. Understanding the genetic basis of channel diversity.

7. Understanding how the patch clamp technique and the reconstitution of channels in artificial bilayers can be used to study channel function.

■ *COMPLETION PROBLEMS*

1. Lipid bilayers are _____ to ions.

2. The lipids of cell membranes do not mix with water because they are _____.

3. Ion channels can be classified into four types: _____-gated, _____-gated, _____-gated, and _____-gated.

4. Because ion channels are _____ for specific ion species, they can be used to generate specific electrical signals.

5. The carrier model of selective membrane permeability is not supported by the high _____ of ions across the membrane during electrical signals.

6. An important aspect of the selectivity of ion channels is their ability to strip the _____ from ions as they enter the aqueous pore by substituting weak chemical bonds (electrostatic interactions) with _____ groups that line the walls of the channel.

7. The _____ technique can be used to measure the unitary ionic currents associated with the opening of single ion channels.

8. The unitary conductance of ion channels has been measured to be in the range of tens of _____.

9. For some ion channels, like those formed by gramicidin A, the ionic current through the channel varies with membrane _____ in a linear fashion, i.e., the channel behaves like a simple _____, and its behavior can be described by _____ law.

10. All ion channels are integral membrane proteins with an _____ that spans the entire width of the membrane.

11. Integral membrane proteins like ion channels often have several alpha helical regions of 15–20 _____ amino acids that span the membrane. Often, ion channels consist of two or more identical or different _____.

12. Ion channels of a particular type, e.g., voltage-gated channels, share strong sequence _____, which indicates that these sequences have been conserved through evolution for particular _____.

13. In voltage-gated channels, strongly conserved membrane-spanning alpha helixes, containing positively charged amino acids in every third position, have been proposed to serve as voltage _____.

14. Immunocytochemistry, chimeric channels, and _____ have all been used to probe channel structure and function at the molecular level.

15. The flux of ions through ion channels is passive, meaning it requires no expenditure of _____.

16. Some cation channels are selective for one ion species, while others allow all _____ usually present in the extracellular fluid (i.e., Na^+, K^+, Mg^{2+}, and Ca^{2+}) to pass.

17. The direction of the ion flux is determined by the _____ and _____ driving forces.

18. The net electrochemical driving force determining the movements of ions through channels is determined by the _____ across the membrane and the _____ of the permeant ion across the membrane.

19. For some channels, current is not a linear function of driving force; such channels are said to _____.

20. At high ion concentrations the current through channels tends to _____; this phenomenon reflects the _____ of ions to polar groups in the channel pore.

21. Because the dissociation constants of ions are small, on the order of _____, the ions typically stay bound in the channel for less than _____, leading to the very high conduction rates necessary for rapid changes in _____ during signaling.

22. Channel blockers operate by _____ to sites in the channel's aqueous pore. If these blockers are charged, their ability to block channel function will be _____-sensitive.

23. Common cations like _____, _____, and _____ can act as channel blockers by binding in and thus occupying space in the channel pore.

24. Nongated channels are always _____ and contribute to the _____ membrane potential.

25. Gated channels open and close by changes in the _____ of the channel proteins.

26. Some channels are gated by the binding of chemical _____, such as neurotransmitters or hormones, while other channels are gated by _____ or _____

27. Voltage-gated channels can exist in several conformational states: closed and _____, open (_____), closed and _____ (refractory).

28. Energy is transferred to ion channels by the _____ of ligands, the mechanical _____ of the membrane, or the _____ field across the membrane, to effect the conformational changes associated with gating.

29. The opening of ion channels is very rapid, taking less than _____, and the sudden opening of several channels gives rise

to the step-like changes in channel current observed with the _____ technique.

30. Ligand-gated channels can enter a refractory state upon prolonged exposure to the ligand in a process known as _____.

31. Some voltage-gated channels also enter refractory states following _____, in a process known as _____. These processes are known in many types of channels to be controlled by different _____ of the channel proteins. For other voltage-gated channels inactivation is dependent on _____ influx.

32. Some drugs and toxins block ligand-gated channels by binding to the same site as the ligand. Such _____ binding can be low energy and _____ or high energy and _____. Other blocking substances interfere with the gating mechanisms of ligand-, stretch-, or voltage-gated channels by binding to different sites in a _____ manner.

33. Channels often occur as a series of closely related forms (_____) that vary in their sensitivity to various activators or _____. Channel variants can be expressed at different _____ stages, in different cell _____, or in different _____ of a given cell.

34. The existence of different types of channels with different properties makes it possible to design _____ drugs that can activate or block channels in particular regions of the nervous system, thus minimizing _____.

35. Three gene families encode most of the known ion channels described so far. One family encodes the _____ channels, another the _____ channels, and the third encodes the _____channels. Ion channels within a family have substantially similar _____ sequences. Each family is thought to have arisen from a common ancestral gene by _____ and _____.

36. In addition to controlling the rapid changes in _____ necessary for electrical signaling, ion channels control _____ influx, which in turn regulates many metabolic processes in the cell and also triggers _____ release.

■ SYNTHETIC QUESTIONS AND QUANTITATIVE PROBLEMS

1. Would you expect the binding site for the permeant ion in the aqueous pore of a cation channel that allows the ion to shed its waters of hydration to contain positively or negatively charged amino acid residues? Why?

2. How would you determine the conductance of individual acetylcholine-gated channels like the one illustrated in Figure 7–5 in the textbook?

3. Certain ligand-gated cation channels allow Ca^{2+} to flow through them, whereas different but related channels gated by the same ligand do not. Alteration of a single positively charged amino acid in a membrane-spanning region of one of the channel's subunits renders that channel, which normally does not flux Ca^{2+}, able to do so. Provide a plausible explanation.

4. Two drugs, A and B, bind relatively weakly to a certain ligand-gated channel, and both block its response to low concentrations of the gating ligand. When the ligand is presented in high concentration in the presence of each drug, the blockage of drug A but not drug B is relieved. Explain.

5. All of the voltage-gated cation channels described (at the molecular level) to date open in response to depolarization and derive from the same gene family but differ in their ion selectivity. What regions of the channel proteins would you expect to be conserved across the members of the family, and what regions would you expect to be divergent?

Answers

▨ *COMPLETION PROBLEMS*

1. impermeable

2. hydrophobic

3. voltage; ligand; mechanically; non

4. selective

5. rates of transfer

6. waters of hydration; charged

7. patch clamp

8. picosiemens

9. potential; resistor; ohm's

10. aqueous pore

11. hydrophobic; subunits

12. similarity; functions

13. sensors

14. site-directed mutagenesis

15. metabolic energy

16. cations

17. electrostatic; diffusional

18. electrical potential difference; concentration gradient

19. rectify

20. saturate; binding

21. 100 mm; 1 ms; membrane potential

22. binding; voltage

23. Mg^{2+}; Ca^{2+}; Na^+

24. open; resting

25. conformational state

26. ligands; voltage; mechanical stretch

27. activatable; active; nonactivatable

28. binding; deformation; electrical

29. 10 ms; patch clamp

30. desensitization

31. activation; inactivation; subunits; Ca^{2+}

32. competitive; reversible; irreversible; noncompetitively

33. isoforms; blockers; developmental; types; regions

34. specific; side effects

35. voltage-gated; ligand-gated; gap-junction; amino acid; duplication; divergence

36. membrane potential; Ca^{2+}; transmitter

SYNTHETIC QUESTIONS AND QUANTITATIVE PROBLEMS

1. One would expect the site to contain negatively charged amino acid residues (or polar amino acids with a strongly negative pole), so that the site could bind weakly to the cation by electrostatic interactions and thus substitute for the weak bond between the cation and the negative polar end of its water of hydration.

2. The single-channel currents are measured with a patch clamp at a series of different membrane (patch) potentials. The amplitudes of the single-channel currents are then plotted as a function of the membrane (patch) potential. The slope of the straight line would be the conductance of a single channel. Ohm's law states the $g = \Delta I/\Delta V$.

3. The positive amino acid probably is exposed in the channel pore and obstructs the movement of the divalent cation Ca^{2+} past it at least partially by electrostatic repulsion. Removal of this electrostatic obstacle allows divalent Ca^{2+} to pass.

4. A binds in a competitive fashion, i.e., to the same binding site as the activating ligand, and thus its blockage can be alleviated by competion for this site by binding with an excess of activating ligand. B binds noncompetitively to a site on the channel where the activating ligand does not bind, but where it can interfere with channel gating. Because the activating ligand does not compete for the binding site of B, elevating its concentration does not alleviate B's blockage.

5. The voltage sensor regions are likely to be conserved, because these act similarly in all channels. The protein segments lining the channel pore are likely to vary as actions in the pore account for a channel's selectivity for specific ion species.

8

Membrane Potential

Overview

The resting membrane potential results from the separation of ionic charges across the nerve cell membrane. This separation of charge in turn results from the asymmetric distribution of different ion species across the membrane (ion concentration gradients) and from the selective permeability of the membrane (resting ion channels). Sodium is more highly concentrated on the outside of the cell and K^+ on the inside, and their concentration gradients are maintained by the tireless action of the sodium-potassium pump, which derives the energy necessary for the active transport of ions against their concentration gradients from the hydrolysis of ATP. Impermeant organic anions are highly concentrated inside the cell. Chloride is passively distributed across the membrane in many neurons or is held slightly below its equilibrium concentration internally by the action of chloride pumps.

A steady state is achieved in which the flux of K^+ out of the cell is balanced by the flux of Na^+ into the cell. The flux of Cl^- and the electrogenic current of the sodium-potassium pump play minor roles. In living neurons that are metabolically maintaining their ion concentration gradients, this balance occurs when the inside of the cell is negative and quite close to the K^+ equilibrium potential. Here, the electrochemical driving force (the sum of the electrical driving force and the chemical driving force due to the concentration gradient) on K^+ is small but the resting permeability to K^+ is high, which leads to a moderate steady leak of K^+ ions out of the cell. In

61

contrast, the electrochemical driving force on Na^+ is large while the resting permeability to Na^+ is small, leading to an equivalent steady inward leak of Na^+.

The membrane of the nerve cell at rest can be represented by an electrical equivalent model, and this model can be used to calculate the membrane potential whenever it is not changing. In the model the membrane lipid bilayer is represented by capacitance, the ion channels by ion-specific conductances (resistances), the ion concentration gradients by ion-specific batteries, and the sodium-potassium pump by a current generator.

Objectives

1. Understanding how the separation of charge across the nerve cell membrane leads to a resting membrane potential.

2. Understanding how the selectivity of a variety of resting ion channels leads to the overall selective permeability of the cell membrane.

3. Understanding how concentration gradients for ions in combination with selective membrane permeability leads to the separation of charge and thus to the resting membrane potential.

4. Understanding the role of the sodium-potassium pump in maintaining ion concentration gradients across the cell membrane and the contribution of its electrogenic current to the resting membrane potential.

5. Understanding the difference between the equilibrium model of the resting membrane potential for the glial cell (permeable only to K^+) and the steady state model for the neuron (permeable to several ion species but predominantly to K^+).

6. Understanding the application of the Nernst and Goldman equations.

7. Understanding the equivalent circuit model for the resting neuronal membrane and its use in calculating V_m when V_m is unchanging.

8. Understanding the functional equivalents of the membrane capacitance (lipid bilayer), conductances (ion channels), batteries (ion concentration gradients), and current generator (sodium-potassium pump) in an electrical equivalent model.

■ *MATCHING PROBLEMS*

1. Resting membrane potential

2. Cations

3. Less negative membrane potential

4. Increase in charge separation across membrane

5. Electrotonic potential

6. Passive response

7. Threshold

8. Diffusion

9. Membrane permeability

10. Membrane conductance

11. Resting channels

12. Nernst Potential

13. Electrochemical driving force

14. Maintenance of ionic concentration gradients

15. Dissipation of ionic gradients

16. Metabolic energy for ion pumping

A. hyperpolarization

B. nongated ion channels

C. regenerative activation of voltage-gated ion channels

D. equilibrium potential

E. sodium-potassium pump

F. ion channels

G. Ohm's law

H. transient reversal of membrane potential

I. passive response

J. resistor (conductor)

K. measured in amperes

L. current generator

M. charge separation across (potential) membrane

N. concentration gradient

O. current flow through nongated ion channels

P. positively charged ions

17. No net ionic flux and main-
    tenance of concentration
    gradients by ion pumping

Q. two conductors separated by an
   insulating material

18. Action potential

R. battery

19. Electrical equivalent of mem-
    brane conductance

S. no net ionic current and maintenance of charged batteries by
   a current generator

20. Electrical equivalent of ionic
    concentration gradient

T. charged capacitor

21. Electrical equivalent of charge
    separation by the cell's lipid
    bilayer

U. measured in volts

22. Electrical equivalent of
    sodium-potassium pump

V. sum of chemical force (potential), i.e., concentration gradient, and electrical (electrostatic)
   force (potential)

23. Capacitance

W. cell death

24. $V = IR = I/G$

X. depolarization

25. Electrical current

Y. measured in farads

26. Electrical potential

Z. ATP

27. Capacitor

AA. steady state

28. Electrical equivalent of
    steady state

BB. channel proteins

◼ SYNTHETIC QUESTIONS AND QUANTITATIVE PROBLEMS

1. Suppose you penetrate a perfectly spherical neuron with current injection and voltage recording electrodes. The resting membrane potential of the cell is –60 mV, and it is 60 μm in diameter (radius = 30 μm). Assume that, like most animal cells, the lipid bilayer of the cell has a capacitance of 1/μF per cm².

   (a) Draw the equivalent circuit of the neuron and electrodes, assuming it to have a passive membrane, and include the membrane potential "battery." Label the components and identify which constituents of the membrane give rise to the resistive and capacitive properties of the equivalent circuit.

   (b) How much charge is stored on the total membrane capacitance (and on the membrane capacitance per square micrometer) at the resting membrane potential of –60 mV? How much charge must be redistributed on the total membrane capacitance to achieve a membrane potential of +40 mV? If the total concentration of cations in the cell is 150 mM — which translates into a concentration of 9×10^{19} cations per cm³, where 1 cm³ is equivalent to 1 ml — by what percentage will the configuration change, if enough cations are redistributed to bring the membrane potential to +40 mV?

      HINTS: The surface area of a sphere is given by the formula $A = 4\pi a^2$, where a is the radius, and the volume of a sphere is given by the formula $V = 4/3\ \pi a^3$. There are 6.2×10^{18} unit charges per coulomb.

2. For a neuronal cell body at 25°C you find that $[K^+]_{out}$ = 20 mM, $[K^+]_{in}$ = 400 mM, $[Na^+]_{out}$ = 400 mM, $[Na^+]_{in}$ = 40 mM. You then measure the permeability ratio for Na⁺ and K⁺, P_{Na}/P_K, and find it to be 0.1. Ignoring Cl⁻, rearrange the Goldman equation (Equation 6, page 140 in the textbook) so that you can compute the resting membrane potential of the neuron from these values and then perform the calculation. What value would the membrane potential reach if P_{Na}/P_K were 1?

3. For a neuronal cell body at 25°C you find that $[K^+]_{out}$ = 20 mM, $[K^+]_{in}$ = 400 mM, $[Na^+]_{out}$ = 440 mM, $[Na^+]_{in}$ = 50 mM, $[Cl^-]_{out}$ = 540 mM, and $[Cl^-]_{in}$ –60 mM. You then measure the conductance for each of these ions and find g_K = 0.75 μs, g_{Na} = 0.1 μs, and g_{Cl} = 0.3 μs.

(a) Compute the equilibrium potential for each ion.

(b) Using the equivalent circuit model of the nerve cell membrane, compute the resting potential of the neuron.

(c) Which ion is closest to being at equilibrium? Give a plausible explanation for why this is so.

(d) What would be the effect on the resting potential of a twofold increase in g_{Na} or a twofold increase in g_K?

4. On the planet ZicZac, life in the dilute primordial sea has not progressed past the evolution of unicellular organisms. The top predators in the primordial sea are huge amoebae-like unicells, called tyranocytes, that prey on herds of helpless flagellated photosynthetic Euglena-like unicells of various species, all called foddercytes. An advanced species of foddercyte, the polyseracyte, has evolved an effective defense mechanism; when it feels the clammy pseudopod of a tyranocyte, it transiently everts hundreds of spike-like spines that render it a bristly meal indeed. The sea is mainly a solution of NaCl with a bit of $Ca(HCO_3)_2$ and is always at 25°C due to geothermal warming. Specifically, the external concentrations of Na^+ and Cl^- are 25 mM; those of Ca^{2+} and HCO_3^- are 1 mM.

  A successful manned mission to ZicZac affords you the opportunity to study these organisms in your lab here on earth. You make the following observations. The membrane of the polyseracyte is permeable to Na^+ but also a bit permeable to Cl^-, i.e., the membrane contains a high density of resting Na^+ channels and a low density of resting Cl^- channels. The membrane is impermeable to HCO_3^- and Ca^{2+} has a very low but finite permeability. Expressed as conductances, these permeability differences work out to a conductance ratio, g_{Cl}/g_{Na}, of .05 ($g_{Na} = 1 \times 10^{-6}$ S, $g_{Cl} = 0.05 \times 10^{-6}$ S). The membrane also contains a pump that is electroneutral and pumps both Na^+ and Cl^- into the cell so that the internal concentration of both Na^+ and Cl^- are 250 mM. There is a similar but outwardly directed calcium–HCO_3^- pump that maintains the internal concentration of these ions at 0.001 mM. Compute the equilibrium potentials for Na^+, Cl^-, and Ca^{2+}. Draw an equivalent circuit representation of the polyseracyte membrane, including conductances for Na^+, Cl^-, and Ca^{2+} — don't forget the membrane capacitance. Using this model and ignoring any possible small contribution from Ca^{2+}, compute the resting potential of the polyseracyte. Redraw the equivalent circuit model with the Na^+ and Cl^- conductances lumped together as a resting or leak conductance. (Keep your answers and work handy, because we will explore the planet ZicZac further in future problems.)

5. Use the computer program APSIM to explore how the resting potential is affected by changes in external ion concentrations. Set the simulation mode to Passive Membrane. You can now simulate the effects of changes in external ion concentration by editing the concentration values for Na^+, K^+, and Cl^- (use the Ionic Concentration Option in Edit Menu). When the external ion concentration is changed, the concentration ratio is changed, so the equilibrium (reversal) potential shifts according to the Nernst equation. If you make a mistake, press the Default button and start over.

6. Using APSIM, explore how the resting potential is affected by the resting conductances to Na^+, K^+, and Cl^-. Set the simulation mode to Passive Membrane. You can now simulate the effects of changes in the resting conductances to Na^+, K^+, or Cl^- by editing the maximal conductance values for Na^+, K^+, and Cl^-. If you make a mistake, select Passive Membrane again and start over.

ANSWERS

▰ *MATCHING PROBLEMS*

1. M.

2. P.

3. X.

4. A.

5. I.

6. O.

7. C.

8. N.

9. BB.

10. F.

11. B.

12. D.

13. V.

14. E.

15. W.

16. Z.

17. AA.

18. H.

19. J.

20. R.

21. T.

22. L.

23. Y.

24. G.

25. K.

26. U.

27. Q.

28. S.

SYNTHETIC QUESTIONS AND QUANTITATIVE PROBLEMS

1. (a) The membrane capacitance can be associated with the nonconductive lipid constituents of the membrane, while the resistance (or conductance) is associated with ion channels, which are integral membrane proteins.

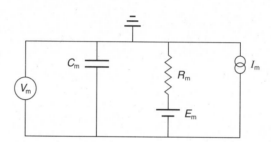

(b) The charge stored on the membrane capacitance is given by the expression $Q_t = C_t V_m$, where Q_t is the total membrane charge, C_t is the total membrane capacitance, and V_m is the membrane potential. The total surface area of the cell is 1.1×10^{-4} cm^2 and its total capacitance is thus 1.1×10^{-10} F. Thus, at a resting potential of –60 mV, the amount of charge stored on the total membrane capacitance is 6.6×10^{-12} coulombs (C), or, since there are 6.2×10^{18} charges per coulomb, 4.1×10^7 charges. Since the surface area of the cell is 1.1×10^4 cm^2, this number translates into 3.7×10^{11} charges per cm^2 or 3.7×10^3 charges per μm^2. Moving the membrane potential to +40 mV involves a voltage change of 100 mV, necessitating a redistribution of 6.8×10^7 charges on the total membrane capacitance. Since the volume of the cell is 1.1×10^{-7} cm^3, and at rest there are 9×10^{19} cations per cm^3 in the cell, the cell contains 9.9×10^{12} cations, so the change of membrane potential to +40 mV will change the internal concentration of cations by $6.8 \times 10^7/9.9 \times 10^{12} \times 100\%$, or less than 1 part in ten thousand.

2. At 25°C $RT/F = 25$ and the conversion factor from natural log to log base ten is 2.3. Rearranging the Goldman equation is simple if we set $\alpha = P_{Na}/P_K$ and divide both the numerator and the denominator of the right side of the equation by P_K. We obtain:

$$V_m = 58 \log \frac{[K^+]_{out} + \alpha[Na^+]_{out}}{[K^+]_{in} + \alpha[Na^+]_{in}}$$

Substituting 0.1 for α yields –48 mV for the resting potential. Substituting 1 for α yields –1 mV for the resting potential. This last calculation supports the intuitive notion that if the permeability to Na^+ and K^+ were equal there would be no resting potential.

3. (a) $E_K = -75$ mV, $E_{Na} = +55$ mV, $E_{Cl} = -55$ mV. The Nernst equilibrium potential for an ion species at 25°C is given by the equation $E_a = RT/ZF \ln([a]_o/[a]_i) = 58/Z \log([a]_o/[a]_i)$, where Z is the charge on the ion.

   (b) The membrane potential at rest $V_m = -58$ mV. Remember $V_m = (E_a g_a + E_b g_b + ...) / (g_a + g_b + ...)$.

   (c) Cl^- is closest to equilibrium at $V_m = -58$ mV, probably because g_{Cl} is relatively high and Cl^- is not pumped to maintain a concentration gradient in opposition to V_m.

   (d) For a twofold increase in g_K, V_m moves to –65 mV, while for a twofold increase in g_{Na}, V_m moves to –49 mV.

4. $E_{Cl} = 58$ mV (remember that for Cl⁻, $Z = -1$)

    $E_{Na} = -58$ mV

    $E_{Ca} = 87$ mV (remember that for Ca²⁺, $Z = 2$)

    $V_m = -52$ mV

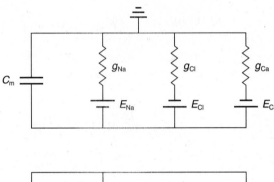

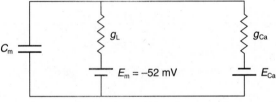

9

Local Signaling: Passive Electrical Properties of the Neuron

Overview

The membrane and processes of neurons have resistive and capacitive properties. The resistance of the membrane is inversely related to the resting ion channels, which permit the flow of ions across the membrane; because the ion channels are limited in their unit conductance and density, membranes have relatively high resistances to the flow of ionic current and thus act as insulators. The capacitance of membranes derives from the lipid bilayer, which permits the separation of charge between the internal conducting fluid (cytoplasm) and the extracellular fluid. This separation of charge, or capacitance, is large for two reasons: (1) the bilayer is thin (4 nm) and therefore permits close apposition of the two conducting fluids on either side of the membrane, and (2) the surface area of the membrane is extensive. Because the resistance and capacitance of membranes act in parallel, membranes can be considered leaky capacitors. The effect of capacitance is to delay any change in membrane potential; charge must be redistributed on the membrane, which takes time. The membrane time constant, τ, is a direct indicator of this delaying effect.

Neuronal processes — axons and dendrites — also have significant axial resistance to the current flow, which increases with their length and decreases with the diameter of the cytoplasmic core. The spread of electrotonic potentials along processes is determined by the efficiency of axial current flow, which in turn is determined by both the axial resistance and the membrane resistance. The lower the axial resistance the more current flows axially; the higher the membrane resistance the less current is lost from axial flow. These two factors determine the length constant, λ, of the process, which is a direct indicator of the efficiency of electrotonic conduction.

The passive electrical properties of neurons thus determine the efficiency of spatial and temporal summation of synaptic potentials in the neuron's dendritic tree. Because of these properties, neurons rely on a regenerative mechanism, the action potential, for long-distance signaling. Nevertheless, the cell's passive electrical properties limit the conduction velocity of the action potentials.

Objectives

1. Understanding how the resistive and capacitive properties of neurons influence electrical signaling.

2. Understanding the physical bases of the membrane time constant and the length constant.

3. Understanding how the membrane time constant affects the conduction velocity of action potentials and the temporal summation of synaptic potentials.

4. Understanding how the length constant limits the spread of electrotonic potentials, thus necessitating action potentials for long-distance signaling, and limits spatial summation of synaptic potentials.

5. Understanding how myelin increases conduction velocity by reducing membrane capacitance and thus the membrane time constant.

■ *COMPLETION PROBLEMS*

1. For an idealized spherical neuron with no processes, the input resistance, R_{in}, depends on both the _____ of resting ion channels in the membrane and the _____ of the membrane, i.e., the size of the cell.

2. The specific membrane resistance, R_m, is the resistance of a unit _____ of membrane. Thus, it is a property of the particular membrane in question and not its size, and depends on the density of _____ and their unit _____. The units of R_m are _____.

3. If two neurons have identical membranes and thus identical R_m, but neuron A has twice the diameter of neuron B, then R_{in} for neuron A will have _____ that of B.

4. When we consider real neurons with processes, then the simple relations between R_{in} and R_m no longer pertain and we must also consider the _____ resistance.

5. To alter the voltage across the capacitor requires that _____ be deposited or removed from the capacitor.

6. The cell membrane acts like a _____ capacitor that is charged at rest. To change the membrane potential resulting from this charge separation, we must redistribute charge on the _____.

7. Membrane capacitance is directly proportional to the _____ of the membrane (the larger the _____ the more _____ can be stored at a given voltage) and inversely proportional to the distance between the _____.

8. For cells A and B of question 3, the capacitance of cell A will be _____ that of cell B.

9. The membrane is called a leaky capacitor because it has a finite resistance due to _____ as well as capacitance due to the _____. The resistance and capacitance act in _____ since the total membrane current (I_m) can flow through ion channels (ionic current, I_i) or simply change the charge distribution across the membrane (i.e., capacitive current, I_c, can flow into and out of the membrane capacitor). $I_m =$ _____ + _____.

10. The redistribution of charge on the membrane _____ the rate at which the membrane potential can change in response to current. In electrical terms we say that the membrane capacitance _____ changes in V_m.

11. Because of the parallel nature of the membrane resistance and capacitance, the total current (I_m) injected during an experiment like the one in Figure 9–1 in the textbook only equals the current through the ion channels, (i.e., through the membrane _____) when the membrane capacitance is fully _____ by the current pulse (i.e., once a steady state voltage is achieved). Under these conditions, I_m = _____, and we can compute R_{in} as $\Delta V_0 /$_____, where ΔV_0 is the steady state voltage change.

12. The membrane time constant, τ, is the time it takes for the voltage change to achieve _____% of the steady state value, and can be computed as the product of the _____ and _____ of the membrane.

13. Electrotonic potentials _____ in amplitude with _____ as they spread along an axon or dendrite.

14. The greater the length of a neuronal process, the _____ the axial resistance of its cytoplasmic core. The larger the diameter of a neuronal process, the _____ the axial resistance of its cytoplasmic core.

15. The greater the length of a neuronal process, the _____ the resistance of its total membrane. The larger the diameter of a neuronal process, the _____ the resistance of its total membrane.

16. When expressed in terms of the axial resistance of a unit length of the cytoplasmic core (r_a) and the membrane resistance of a unit length of the process cylinder (r_m), the membrane length constant (λ) = _____. The length constant represents the distance over which the steady state amplitude of an electrotonic potential is attenuated by _____%.

17. Because the attenuation of an electrotonic potential with distance is _____, electrotonic potentials die out completely at a distance of 10λ. Typical values for λ of neuronal processes lie between _____ and _____ mm.

18. When expressed in terms of the specific membrane resistance R_m (measured in units of _____), the specific resistivity of the

cytoplasm R_a (measured in units of _____), and the process radius (a), λ = _____. This expression shows that λ is _____ to the square root of the process radius.

19. Because the total membrane resistance of a cylindrical process decreases as the _____ of the radius of the process and the total axial resistance decreases as the _____ of the radius of the process, all other things otherwise being equal, a large-diameter process will be _____ efficient for electrotonic conduction than a small-diameter process.

20. The time it takes for an electrotonic potential to reach its steady state value as it spreads along a neural process is determined by both the _____ and the _____ per unit length of the process. Thus, the time delays associated with passive spread varies inversely with the product _____. These delays affect the _____ of action potentials; the passive spread of depolarization from an action potential _____ the attainment of threshold in adjacent regions of the axon.

21. Increasing the diameter of the axon core increases conduction velocity, because the axial resistance of a unit length of the axon, r_a, decreases in proportion to the _____ of the axon radius, while the membrane capacitance of a unit length of the axon, c_m, increases as the _____ of the axon radius.

22. Myelination increases the separation of the cytoplasmic core from the extracellular fluid and thus increases conduction velocity because it reduces _____.

23. The regularly distributed nodes of Ranvier in a myelinated axon serve as points where the action potential is periodically _____. Because the action potential jumps quickly from node to node, the conduction is called _____.

24. Demyelinating diseases can _____ and even _____ the conduction of action potentials.

25. A neuron with a long time constant has a greater power of _____ summation of synaptic potentials at the trigger zone. The short length constant of dendrites limits the extent of _____ summation of synaptic potentials and thus forces the neuron to have a relatively compact trigger zone.

◼ SYNTHETIC QUESTIONS AND QUANTITATIVE PROBLEMS

1. Suppose you penetrate a perfectly spherical neuron with current injection and voltage recording electrodes. The resting membrane potential of the cell is –60 mV, and it is 60 μm in diameter (a = 30 μm).

   (a) Suppose you inject square pulses (20, 40, and 100 ms in duration) of hyperpolarizing current into such a cell, and generate the voltage and current records presented in the figure below. What is the time constant τ of the cell? What is its input resistance R_{in} and input capacitance C_{in}?

   (b) If you could in god-like fashion increase the radius of the cell by the factor 2 while keeping the specific membrane resistance and capacitance constant, what effect would this minor miracle have on the input resistance R_{in} and time constant τ of the cell? Why?

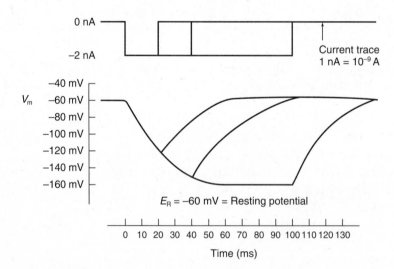

Figure 9–1

2. You penetrate a squid giant axon with a series of microelectrodes for current injection (*stim*) and voltage recording (*rec*) as shown below.

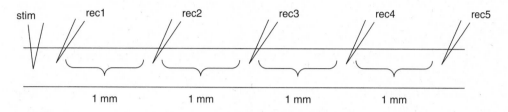

Figure 9–2

Assume that the resting membrane potential of the axon is –60 mV and that the membrane contains only resting (leakage channels).

(a) Draw the equivalent circuit of the axon excluding the membrane potential "battery." Label the components, and identify which constituents of the membrane or cytoplasm give rise to the resistive and capacitive properties of the equivalent circuit.

(b) You inject a square pulse of hyperpolarizing current at *stim* that has a duration greater than 10 times τ as measured at *rec 1*. Describe the decline of the steady state voltage reached during the pulse with distance from *rec 1* in terms of the membrane resistance per unit length (cm) of axon membrane, r_m, and the resistance of a unit length (cm) of axon core, r_a, and in terms of the specific resistance of the membrane, R_m, the axon core, R_a, and the axon's radius a. Suppose that $R_a = 30$ Ω-cm, $R_m = 600$ Ω-cm^2, and $a = 0.04$ mm. Calculate the length contstant, λ. Draw the voltage records from each recording site given an initial steady state hyperpolarization at 50 mV of *rec 1*. Be as quantitative as possible by assigning approximate values to the equilibrium voltage recorded at each site. How does the time course of the approach to the equilibrium voltage change with distance from *rec 1*?

3. (a) Compare the electrical and chemical properties of the nodal and internodal regions of a myelinated axon. Include with your answer a diagram of a low-magnification electron micrograph of a longitudinal section through both regions (see Figure 3–4 in the textbook, p. 49).

(b) What difference would you expect to see in the distances between nodes in large and small axons? Why?

(c) What alterations in the propagation characteristics of axons would you expect in patients suffering from a demyelinating disease? Explain.

4. Use the computer program APSIM to determine the input resistance R_{in}, time constant τ, and input capacitance C_{in} of the axon. Set the simulation mode to Active Membrane. Inject a hyperpolarizing pulse (30 ms long, -10 µA in amplitude) into the axon and use Measure to obtain the values necessary for your calculation. Notice that an action potential is produced upon release from the hyperpolarizing pulse. This phenomenon is called postinhibitory rebound and is due to removal of inactivation from voltage-gated Na^+ channels by the hyperpolarization; see Chapter 10 in the textbook (p. 168).

ANSWERS

■ COMPLETION PROBLEMS

1. density; surface area

2. area; resting channels; conductance; Ω-cm^2

3. one-fourth

4. axial

5. charge

6. leaky; membrane capacitance

7. surface area; area; charge; inside and outside of the membrane

8. four times

9. ion channels; lipid bilayer; parallel; I_i; I_c

10. reduces; delays

11. resistance; charged; I_i; I_m

12. 63; resistance; capacitance

13. decrease; distance

14. greater; smaller

15. smaller; smaller

16. $\sqrt{(r_m/r_a)}$; 63

17.   exponential; 0.1; 1

18. Ω-cm^2; Ω-cm; $\sqrt{(aR_m/2R_a)}$; proportional

19.   first power; square; more

20.   membrane resistance; capacitance; RC; conduction velocity; delays

21.   square; first power

22.   capacitance

23.   regenerated; saltatory

24.   slow; block

25.   temporal; spatial

■ SYNTHETIC QUESTIONS AND QUANTITATIVE PROBLEMS

1. (a) $\tau = 20$ ms, $R_{in} = 50$ MΩ, $C_{IN} = 0.4$ nF. Remember that $R_{in} = \Delta V_0/I_m$, where ΔV_0 is the equilibrium voltage attained during the current pulse and I_m is the current injected, i.e., the total membrane current, and that $\tau = R_{in}C_{in}$ and $\Delta V_t = \Delta V_0 (1e^{-t/\tau})$. τ and ΔV_0 can be measured directly from the records in Figure 9–1 and R_{in} and C_{in} calculated.

    (b)   Since for a spherical cell, $R_{in} = R_m/A = R_m/4\tau a^2$, then if the radius is doubled, R_{in} will be quartered. Since for a spherical cell, $C_{in} = C_m A = C_m (4\tau a^2)$, then if the radius is doubled, C_{in} will be quadrupled. Since R_{in} is quartered and C_{in} is quadrupled, the time constant, τ, will remain unchanged ($\tau = R_{in}C_{in}$).

2. (a) The membrane capacitance can be associated with the nonconductive lipid constituents of the membrane, while the resistance (or conductance) is associated with resting ion channels, which are integral membrane proteins. The axial resistance is the resistance of the cytoplasm, a complex aqueous solution containing several inorganic ions. These ions are the main current carriers in the cytoplasm.

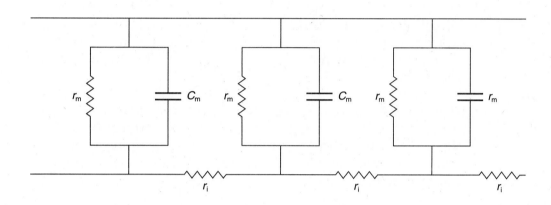

(b) $\lambda = 2$ mm

$$\Delta V = \Delta V_0 \exp(-x/\lambda), \text{ where } \lambda = \sqrt{\frac{r_m}{r_a}} = \sqrt{\frac{aR_m}{2R_a}}$$

ΔV_0 is the steady state voltage attained at the site of current injection, i.e., at *rec 1,* and x is the distance from *rec 1,* the site of current injection. r_m is given in Ω-cm, r_a is given in Ω/cm, R_m is given in Ω-cm^2, and R_a is given in Ω-cm.

(c)

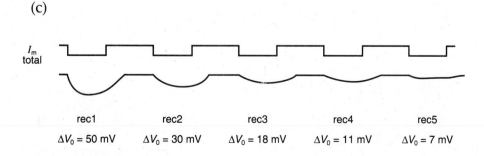

rec1	rec2	rec3	rec4	rec5
$\Delta V_0 = 50$ mV	$\Delta V_0 = 30$ mV	$\Delta V_0 = 18$ mV	$\Delta V_0 = 11$ mV	$\Delta V_0 = 7$ mV

The time necessary to attain the steady state voltage increases with increasing distance.

3. (a) The node has a high density of voltage-gated Na^+ channels, a high membrane capacitance, and a low membrane resistance. The internode has a very low density of voltage-gated Na^+ channels, low membrane capacitance, and a high membrane resistance.

    (b) Small-diameter axons have a smaller internodal distance because they have larger r_a and therefore smaller λ. Thus the electrotronic spread of the depolarization associated with an action potential is limited.

    (c) The conduction velocity of action potentials will slow because of increased membrane capacitance. Failure of transmission may occur because of the patchy distribution of voltage-gated Na^+ channels (essentially located only at the old nodes), and reduced membrane resistance leading to reduced λ.

4. R_{in} = 2.3 kΩ, τ = 2.3 ms, C_{in} = 1 μF.

10

Propagated Signaling:
The Action Potential

Overview

The action potential is used by all animal nervous systems for high-speed long-distance signaling. The basic mechanisms of the action potential were elucidated by the pioneering voltage-clamp studies of A. L. Hodgkin and A. F. Huxley on the squid giant axon. We now know that these basic mechanisms are found in all animals; some variations occur, but within the same basic plan.

In its most basic form, as exemplified in the squid giant axon, the action potential derives from the concerted action of two types of channels: voltage-gated Na^+ and K^+ channels. The voltage-gated Na^+ channels can exist in three different states: resting (functionally closed), activated (functionally open), and inactivated (functionally closed). The resting state is favored by a negative membrane potential and the active state results from depolarization. The active state gives way to the inactivated state. The voltage-gated Na^+ channels lead to the rising phase of the regenerated action potential. Opening and closing of the channels by depolarization leads to further depolarization (inward Na^+ current) and thus more channel openings — a positive feedback relation. Inactivation of voltage-gated Na^+ channels during the course of the action potential contributes to repolarization of the membrane.

Voltage-gated K^+ channels can exist in two different states: resting (functionally closed) and activated (functionally open). The resting state is favored by a negative membrane potential and the active state results from depolarization, but the attainment of the active state upon depolarization is relatively slow compared to voltage-gated Na^+ channels. The voltage-gated K^+ channels contribute to the repolarizing phase of the action potential and the afterpotential. Opening of these channels by depolarization leads to repolarization (outward K^+ current) and thus eventually to the closing of the channels — a negative feedback relation. Action potentials and other regenerative signals in neurons are a variation on one basic plan: voltage-gated Na^+ and Ca^{2+} channels of various types contribute inward current, and voltage-gated K+ channels of various types contribute outward current.

Voltage-gated channels all derive from one gene family, and the detailed study of their molecular structure yields insights into the general mechanisms of ion selectivity, activation, and inactivation.

Objectives

1. Understanding how the voltage clamp allows study of the ionic mechanisms underlying the action potential.

2. Understanding the gating of voltage-gated channels and the role of voltage-gated Na^+ and K^+ channels in generating the action potential in axons.

3. Understanding the diversity of voltage-gated channels, their molecular structures and relatedness, and their molecular mechanisms of action.

■ COMPLETION PROBLEMS

1. The drug _____ blocks voltage-gated Na^+ channels and the drug _____ blocks voltage-gated K^+ channels.

2. When drugs are used to block voltage-gated K$^+$ channels, the total membrane current observed in voltage-clamp currents from a squid giant axon consists of _____, _____, and _____.

3. In a voltage-clamp experiment, because _____ occurs only briefly at the beginning and end of a voltage pulse, it can be eliminated easily by visual inspection.

4. A voltage-clamp is a _____ feedback system.

5. The increases and decreases in Na$^+$ and K$^+$ current seen in voltage-clamp experiments on squid giant axons reflect the opening and closing of _____ of voltage-gated channels.

6. In the squid axon each voltage-gated Na+ channel can exist in three states: _____, _____, and _____.

7. In the squid axon each voltage-gated K$^+$ channel can exist in two states: _____ and _____.

8. In the squid axon voltage-gated Na$^+$ channels exist in a _____ feedback relation with membrane potential.

9. In the squid axon voltage-gated K$^+$ channels exist in a _____ feedback relation with membrane potential.

10. Despite the fact that Na$^+$ conductance through the neuron's membrane increases in a strictly graded manner as depolarization increases, the action potential has a discrete _____ and is _____.

11. The action potential is followed by a brief period of reduced excitability (or _____), which can be divided into two phases: _____ and _____.

12. These periods of reduced excitability are caused by residual _____ of Na$^+$ channels and _____ of K$^+$ channels.

13. The threshold for an action potential can be defined as the specific value of V_m at which the net ionic current ($I_{Na} + I_K + I_l$) just changes from _____ to _____, thus depositing net _____ on the inside of the membrane.

14. Four types of voltage-gated K$^+$ channels are particularly common in nervous systems: _____, _____, _____, and _____ K$^+$ channels.

15. Calcium is unique among ions that flow through ion channels in that its concentration inside the cell is extremely _____, about _____ *M,* so that the amount of Ca^{2+} that enters a cell during normal electrical activity can _____ the internal concentration.

16. Voltage-gated Na^+ channels of the squid axon have two functional gates, an _____ gate and an _____ gate.

17. In nonmyelinated axons the density of voltage-gated Na^+ channels is quite low, ranging in different cell types from _____ to _____ channels per μM^2. Even at the highest density these channels account for less than _____% of the membrane area.

18. In nonmyelinated axons, despite the low density of voltage-gated Na^+ channels, large Na^+ currents flow during _____ because the flux through individual Na^+ channels is quite high, up to _____ Na^+ ions per second.

19. Voltage-gated Na^+ channels select for Na^+ on the basis of _____, _____, and _____ of the ion.

■ *TRUE/FALSE QUESTIONS*
   (If false, explain why)

1. The basic function of the voltage clamp is to interrupt the interaction between the membrane potential and the opening and closing of voltage-gated channels. _____

2. When the membrane potential is held steady in a voltage clamp, the flow of ionic current still redistributes charge on the membrane capacitance. _____

3. The sum of all the current flows through the resting ion channels of a neuronal membrane is called the leakage current, I_l. _____

4. In a typical neuron most of the resting channels are permeable to Na^+. _____

5. In voltage-clamp studies to elucidate the mechanisms of the action potential, Hodgkin and Huxley achieved separation of the inward Na^+ current from the outward K^+ current by changing ions in the bathing solution. _____

6. Both voltage-gated Na^+ and K^+ channels open in response to depolarizing steps, and they do so more rapidly and with higher probability for larger depolarizations. _____

7. Voltage-gated Na^+ channels open more slowly than voltage-gated K^+ channels upon depolarization, and close more slowly upon repolarization. _____

8. Whereas voltage-gated Na^+ channels of the squid axon inactivate during prolonged depolarization, the voltage-gated K^+ channels do not. _____

9. Both inactivation of voltage-gated Na^+ channels and delayed opening of voltage-gated K^+ channels contribute to the repolarization of the action potential. _____

10. During the absolute refractory period an action potential can be triggered but only by depolarizations that are bigger than normal for eliciting an action potential. _____

11. Inactivation of voltage-gated Na^+ channels can be relieved by repolarizing the membrane. _____

12. To relieve the inactivated state of voltage-gated Na^+ channels, the activation gate must close before the inactivation gate can open. _____

13. The nervous systems of mammals express such a rich variety of voltage-gated channels that Hodgkin and Huxley's studies on the mechanisms of the action potential in squid do not apply to the human brain. _____

14. Activation of calcium-sensitive K^+ channels requires a rise in internal Ca^{2+} concentration but not depolarization. _____

15. In general, voltage-gated ion channels are uniformly distributed among the various regions of a neuron. _____

16. A neuron's response to synaptic input will be determined by the distribution and proportions of the various voltage-gated ion channels in the cell's integrative and trigger zones. _____

17. The widest diversity of voltage-gated channels normally exists in the axon of a neuron, not in its input and output regions. _____

18. Calcium that enters through voltage-gated channels can alter the activity of other channels and act as a second messenger to influence other processes in the cell. _____

19. The lower the density of voltage-gated Na^+ channels in an axonal membrane, the faster the action potential will travel, because the membrane leakage resistance is increased. _____

20. The gating current observed in voltage-clamp studies of voltage-gated Na^+ channels represents the movement of Na^+ ions through the channel pore. _____

21. A low pH in the external solution bathing an axon will protinate acidic amino acid residues within the channel pore of voltage-gated Na^+ channels and reduce the conductance of the open channel for Na^+. _____

22. Voltage-gated Na^+, K^+, and Ca^{2+} channels are all members of the same gene family. _____

23. The function of the S4 region of the voltage-gated Na^+, K^+, and Ca^{2+} channels as a voltage sensor is due to its net negative charge despite being a relatively hydrophobic membrane-spanning α-helix. _____

24. The P segment of voltage-gated Na^+, K^+, and Ca^{2+} channels is a largely hydrophobic β-sheet that dips into and out of the membrane and has negatively charged amino acid residues that may line the channel pore of these cation channel. _____

25. Unlike voltage-gated Na^+ and Ca^{2+} channels, voltage-gated K^+ channels have only two membrane-spanning domains or motifs, each consisting of six membrane-spanning regions and a P segment. _____

SYNTHETIC QUESTIONS AND QUANTITATIVE PROBLEMS

1. Identify all the currents indicated (a-f) according to whether they are capacitative current, I_c; leakage current, I_l; voltage-gated Na$^+$ current, I_{Na}; or voltage-gated K$^+$ current, I_K.

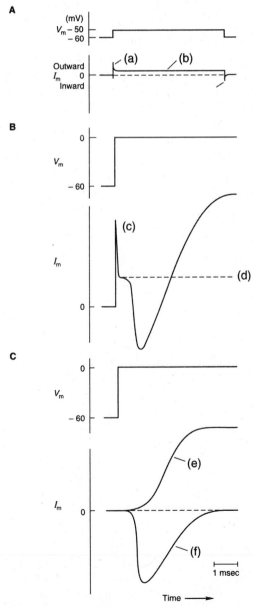

Figure 10–1

2. Fast transient voltage-gated K$^+$ channels (A channels) rapidly inactivate after activation by depolarization. Using the techniques of molecular biology to alter genes and produce mRNAs that can be expressed in cells, it is possible to make cells with A channels missing various parts or having various other changes. A channels produced from A channel proteins lacking the amino terminal end (some 80 amino acids in length) normally located in the cytoplasm will activate normally but do not inactivate. If the first 20 amino acids at the amino terminal end are removed, the same result is observed: no inactivation. If the chain of amino acids following this initial 20 is shortened but the initial 20 (henceforth referred to as the amino ball) are unaltered, inactivation occurs more rapidly than normal. If the chain is lengthened but the ball unaltered, inactivation occurs more slowly than normal. Alteration of positively charged amino acids in the ball to neutral amino acids slows inactivation. In mutant ball-less A channels that do not inactivate, inactivation can be restored by injecting purified ball polypeptide (i.e., the 20 amino acid ball sequence) into the cells expressing the mutant channels.

    What do these experiments tell you about the mechanism of inactivation in A channels and its relation to activation? Removal of the intracellular loop between membrane-spanning domains III and IV of voltage-gated Na$^+$ channels likewise abolishes inactivation without altering activation. Propose a mechanism for inactivation of these voltage-gated Na$^+$ channels.

3. The method of using binding of radiolabeled tetrodotoxin (TTX) to determine the distribution and density of voltage-gated Na$^+$ channels in an axonal membrane is described in the textbook. How would you expect the pattern to be different between myelinated and nonmyelinated axons?

4. The interaction between voltage-gated Na$^+$ channels and membrane potential is characterized in the textbook as a positive feedback relation or regenerative. How would you characterize the interaction between voltage-gated K$^+$ channels and membrane potential?

5. The depolarization that occurs during an action potential when voltage-gated Na$^+$ channels are opened spreads passively to open more voltage-gated Na$^+$ channels. The passive spread of depolarization is bidirectional, but the action potential is propagated in only one direction. Why?

6. What effect would tetrodotoxin (TTX) have on the production of action potentials? What effect would tetraethyl ammonium (TEA) have on the production of action potentials? If either condition would allow for the production of action potentials, how would the action potentials differ from normal action potentials?

7. We return to the laboratory to study once again life from the planet
    ZicZac, so refresh your memory by reviewing Quantitative Problem
    8–4 (p. 67). Remember that when a polyseracyte feels the clammy
    pseudopod of a tyranocyte, it everts hundreds of spike-like spines that
    render it a bristly meal indeed. You now explore the mechanisms by
    which this eversion occurs using intracellular microelectrodes for volt-
    age recording and current injection.

    With these electrodes you are also able to perform voltage-clamp
    experiments of the type done by Hodgkin and Huxley to study the
    action potential in squid axons. You find that, as predicted from your
    analysis reported in Quantitative Problem 4, Chapter 8, the polysera-
    cyte has a resting potential of about –50 mV. Also, whenever the clam-
    my pseudopod of a tyranocyte contacts the polyseracyte, the polyser-
    acyte produces a depolarizing action potential that reaches a mem-
    brane potential at its peak near +50 mV with an afterpotential that
    approaches 55 mV. You find from current injection experiments that
    the membrane is brought to threshold for the generation of the action
    potential at about 35 mV. Every time you elicit an action potential in
    normal extracellular medium you get spine eversion. However, when
    extracellular Ca^{2+} is removed from the medium and replaced by either
    Mg^{2+} or Co^{2+}, which are known to stopper and block earthly Ca^{2+}
    channels, the action potential appears to be unaffected but spike ever-
    sion no longer occurs.

    You perform all further experiments in an extracellular medium
    containing Co^{2+} instead of Ca^{2+}. You find that the peak of the action
    potential is increased (made more positive) when you reduce the
    extracellular concentration of Cl^-, and reduced (less positive) when
    you increase the extracellular concentration of Cl^-. You also find that
    the amplitude of the afterpotential is increased (made more negative)
    when you reduce the extracellular concentration of Na^+, and reduced
    (made less negative) when you increase the extracellular concentra-
    tion of Na+. The new drug nanananabooboolin blocks the action
    potentials and the new drug hobbesisin blocks the afterpotential and
    slows the repolarization.

    (a) Based on your observations, come up with a hypothesis based on
         voltage-gated channels that can account for the action potential.

    (b) You do a voltage-clamp experiment in the presence of hobbesisin.
         From the resting potential (–50 mV) you issue a voltage step com-
         mand to 0 mV. Draw the expected current through voltage-gated
         channels.

    (c) You do a voltage-clamp experiment in the presence of nanananana-
         booboolin. From the resting potential (–50 mV) you issue a volt-
         age step command to 0 mV. Draw the expected current through
         voltage-gated channels.

(d) Based on your observations, come up with a hypothesis based on voltage-gated channels that can account for spike eversion in response to the action potential in normal medium.

8. This question requires you to synthesize information from Chapters 7 through 10 of the textbook. Be sure to review the concepts in Figures 7–4, 7–5 and Box 7–1 in the textbook. Figure 10–2A below shows patch clamp records of single-channel currents through voltage-gated Na^+ channels of the type that underlie action potentials. Figure 10–2B shows patch-clamp records of single-channel currents through voltage-gated K^+ channels of the type that underlie the repolarizing phase of action potentials.

   The records were taken from cultured rat muscle cells in a series of patch-clamp experiments very similar to the procedure used by Hodgkin and Huxley when they did their voltage-clamp studies of the action potential mechanism in squid axons. The difference here is that the currents measured by Hodgkin and Huxley were global (representing the activity of thousands of channels acting in aggregate), whereas the patch-clamp records here represent the activity of one or a few channels isolated in the patch pipette. In the Na^+ channel records the same voltage step is repeated three times (Figure 10–2A),

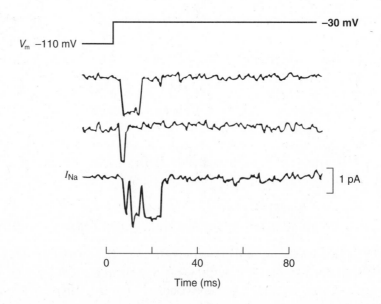

Patch clamp records of voltage-gated Na^+ channels from a cultured rat muscle cell. The patch was held at –110 mV and then stepped to –30 mV. Three successive traces of I_{Na} using this procedure are shown. The time course of the step is indicated above (V_m). Note the current and time scales. Also note that the opening events in each current trace failed to reappear during the time course of the step, i.e. they were limited to the period right at the beginning of the step, which lasted for much longer than shown.

Figure 10–2A

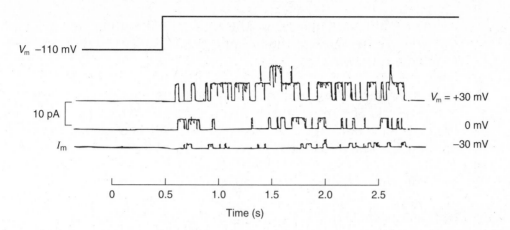

Patch clamp records of voltage-gated K⁺ channels from a cultured rat muscle cell. The patch was held at –110 mV and then stepped to the potential indicated at the right of each current record (I_m). The time course of the step is indicated above (V_m). Note the current and time scales. When calculating single-channel conductance, use the top current trace (V_m = +30 mV) and round the current measurement to the nearest 10 pA.

Figure 10–2B

while in the K⁺ channel records three different step potentials are used (Figure 10–2B). There are several apparent similarities and differences in the records from the Na⁺ and K⁺ channels. Answer the following questions concerning these records.

(a) What is the minimum number of channels in the patch that could account for the K⁺ channel records? Why?

(b) What is the single-channel conductance of the voltage-gated K⁺ and Na⁺ channels? Convince yourself that the flux of ions (ions per second) is indeed large through open voltage-gated Na⁺ channels by calculating this flux for the channels recorded in Figure 10–2A. Assume that E_K is –90 mV and E_{Na} is +50 mV.

(c) Why are the single-channel currents for the K⁺ channels (Figure 10–2B) bigger for the step to +30 mV than for the step to –30 mV?

(d) Other than the size of the single-channel currents, what differences in behavior of the K⁺ channels do you see among the three different voltage steps (Figure 10–2B)? Explain each difference in detail.

(e) Comparing the single-channel currents and the behavior of the Na⁺ and K⁺ channels at steps to –30 mV, identify at least two prominent differences and explain each in terms of the known properties of nerve cells and voltage-gated channels.

(f)   Draw a typical record of the K⁺ channel activity for a step to –60 mV (remember, the holding potential is –110 mV) and justify your drawing.

10. This question reviews material presented in Chapter 7 through 10 of the textbook. Be sure to review Boxes 7–10 and 10–1 in the textbook. Pretend that your experimental system is cultured neurons from the dreaded Georgia opossum.

(a)   You know the following concentrations:

$[K^+]_o = 4$ mM $[K^+]_i = 100$ mM

$[Cl^-]_o = 100$ mM $[Cl^-]_i = 10$ mM

$[Na^+]_o = 100$ mM $[Na^+]_i = 10$ mM

Calculate the equilibrium potential for each ion. Round off your answer to the nearest 5 mV for use in all subsequent questions.

(b)   You know the following conductances for the leakage channels in the membrane:

$g_K = 2$ ms

$g_{Cl} = 0.8$ ms

$g_{Na} = 0.2$ ms

Considering all ions, calculate the resting membrane potential. Round off your answer to the nearest 5 mV for use in all subsequent questions.

(c)   You make the following voltage-clamp records (Figure 10–2C) from one of your neurons. You hold the cell at –60 mV and make a series of depolarizing steps, in increments of 30 mV each, between –30 and +90 mV.

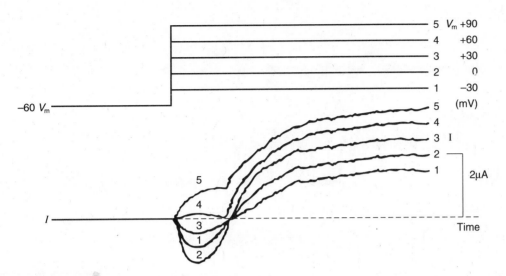

Figure 10C

Adapted from Figure 4–5b from Hodgkin and Huxley, (1952a,b,c; Hodgkin et al, 1952), as reprinted in Levitan and Kaczmarek, *The Neuron: Cell and Molecular Biology*, Oxford University Press: New York, 1991, p 84.

Explain why the early current first increases then decreases with increasing depolarization, while the late current continuously increases with depolarization.

(d) You add a maximal dose of the voltage-gated Na⁺ channel blocker tetrodotoxin (TTX) to the bathing solution and repeat the experiment in (c). Draw the expected current records for the repeat experiment.

(e) Calculate the conductance (g_K) of the population of voltage-gated K⁺ channels opened by the step to 0 mV.

(f) You wash out the TTX from the bathing medium and isolate a single ion channel under a patch-clamp pipette, which contains normal bathing medium. You obtain the following current records for the transpatch potentials indicated (Figure 10–2D).

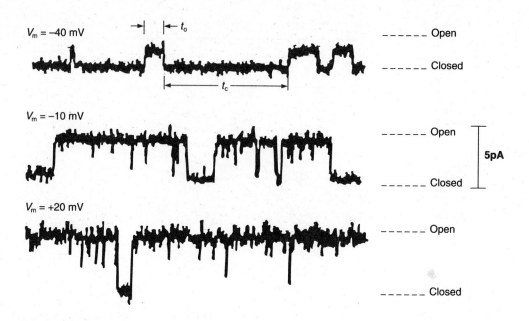

Figure 10D

Adapted from Figure 3–9a from Levitan and Kaczmarek, *The Neuron: Cell and Molecular Biology,* Oxford University Press: New York, 1991, p 70.

Make an educated guess as to the type of channel you have isolated and define as precisely as possible its properties (no need to be quantitative). t_o = time spent in the open state, t_c = time spent in the closed state.

Answers

■ COMPLETION PROBLEMS

1. tetrodotoxin; tetraethyl ammonium

2. I_{Na}; I_C; I_l

3. I_C

4. negative

5. thousands

6. resting; activated; inactivated

7. resting; activated

8. positive

9. negative

10. threshold; all-or-none

11. refractoriness; relative; absolute

12. inactivation; activation

13. outward; inward; positive charge

14. delayed rectifier; Ca^{2+}-sensitive; fast transient; M-type

15. low; 10^{-7}; increase

16. activation; inactivation

17. 35; 100; 1

18. an action potential; 10^7

19. size; charge; energy of hydration

■ *TRUE-FALSE QUESTIONS*

1. True

2. False. When the membrane potential is held steady in a voltage clamp, the flow of ionic current *cannot* redistribute charge on the membrane capacitance.

3. True

4. False. In a typical neuron most of the resting channels are permeable to K^+.

5. True

6. True

7. False. Voltage-gated Na^+ channels open more *rapidly* than voltage-gated K^+ channels upon depolarization, and close more *rapidly* upon repolarization.

8. True

9. True

10. False. During the *relative* refractory period an action potential can be triggered but only by depolarizations that are bigger than normal for eliciting an action potential.

11. True

12. True

13. False. The nervous systems of mammals (including man) express a rich variety of voltage-gated channels whose function has been illuminated by Hodgkin's and Huxley's studies on the mechanisms of the action potential in squid.

14. False. Activation of calcium-sensitive K^+ channels requires *both* a rise in internal Ca^{2+} concentration and depolarization.

15. False. In general, voltage-gated ion channels are *not* uniformly distributed along the various regions of neurons.

16. True

17. False. The widest diversity of voltage-gated channels normally exists in the input and output regions of a neuron, not in its axon.

18. True

19. False. The *higher* the density of voltage-gated Na⁺ channels in an axonal membrane the faster the action potential will travel. The greater channel density allows more current flow through the excited membrane and down the axon core, thus rapidly discharging the capacitance of the unexcited membrane down stream.

20. False. The gating current observed in voltage clamp studies of voltage-gated Na⁺ channels represents the movement of fixed charges in the channel protein from near the inner surface to near the outer surface of the membrane, during gating (activation).

21. True

22. True

23. False. The function of the S4 region of voltage-gated Na⁺, K⁺, and Ca²⁺ channels as a voltage sensor is due to its net *positive* charge despite being a relatively hydrophobic membrane spanning α-helix.

24. True

25. False. Unlike voltage-gated Na⁺ and Ca²⁺ channels, voltage-gated K⁺ channels have only *one* membrane spanning domain or motif, consisting of six membranes spanning regions and a P segment.

◾ SYNTHETIC QUESTIONS AND QUANTITATIVE PROBLEMS

1. See Figure 10–4 in the textbook, p. 166.

2. The experiments are consistent with a model very much like that presented in Figure 7–9C in the textbook (p. 126), where inactivation of the A channel is brought about by a blocking particle ("ball") attached to the inside surface of the channels by a polypeptide ("chain"). When the channel undergoes the conformational change associated with activation, it exposes a negatively charged binding site to which the positive ball binds. The kinetics of this binding is inversely proportional to the length of the chain; if the chain is held close to its activation-generated binding site, it is rapidly attracted to the site. Balls freely mobile in the cytoplasm (dissolved) also have access to this activation-generated binding site.

   In the voltage-gated Na⁺ channel the intracellular loop between domains III and IV may be a ball suspended by two chains, and thus the voltage-gated Na$^+$ channel may have a similar mechanism for inactivation as the A channel.

3. In nonmyelinated axons the voltage-gated Na$^+$ channels would be uniformly distributed at low density. In myelinated axons the voltage-gated Na$^+$ channels should occur at very high density at the nodes of Ranvier and be at extremely low density or nonexistent in the internodes.

4. The interaction between voltage-gated K$^+$ channels and membrane potential can be characterized as a negative feedback relation or self-limiting. Depolarization opens voltage-gated K$^+$ channels, but the effect of this opening (increased K$^+$ conductance) is repolarization of the membrane potential, which in turn leads to the closing of the channels.

5. Even though the passive spread of depolarization associated with an action potential is bidirectional, this depolarization can only reinitiate the action potential at its wave front. In the wake of the action potential the membrane is refractory due to inactivation of voltage-gated Na$^+$ channels and residual activation of voltage-gated K$^+$ channels. Thus, propagation occurs only from the wave front.

6. TTX should make it impossible to produce action potentials regardless of the amount of depolarization, because the voltage-gated Na$^+$ channels that produce the regenerative rising phase of the action potential are blocked by TTX. TEA should make the membrane of a neuron more excitable because voltage-gated K$^+$ channels, which can oppose the regenerative rising phase of the action potential, are blocked. (Remember that threshold is the point where the sum $I_{Na} + I_l + I_K$ turns from outward to inward.) In the presence of TEA the action potential should be propagated and have no afterpotential because the voltage-gated K$^+$ channels, which help repolarize the action potential and produce the afterpotential, are blocked. In the presence of TEA the action potential is repolarized by current through the leakage channels after inactivation of the voltage-gated Na$^+$ channels.

7. (a) The membrane of the polyseracyte contains both voltage-gated Cl$^-$ channels and voltage-gated Na$^+$ channels. Upon depolarization the voltage-gated Cl$^-$ channels activate rapidly while the voltage-gated Na$^+$ channels activate more slowly. The voltage-gated Cl$^-$ channels inactivate upon activation with sustained depolarization (not strictly necessary). The action potential is brought about by the sequential activation of the voltage-gated Cl$^-$ and Na$^+$ channels by depolarization. Upon activation of the Cl$^-$ channels, Cl$^-$ flows out of the cell down its electrochemical

gradient (inward current) depolarizing the cell near E_{Cl} (+59 mV). Inactivation of the Cl⁻ channels and the delayed activation of the Na⁺ channels repolarizes the membrane and produces the after-potential as Na⁺ flows out of the cell down its electrochemical gradient through the open voltage-gated Na⁺ channels (outward current), thus moving the membrane potential toward E_{Na} (–58 mV). Repolarization of the membrane potential then deactivates the voltage-gated Na⁺ channels and the membrane potential is restored to the resting level by current flow through the leakage channels.

(b) Hobbesisin appears to block the voltage-gated Na⁺ channels so they would not contribute to the current observed in the experiment. At a membrane potential of 0 mV one could expect almost complete activation of the voltage-gated Cl⁻ channels, which would produce a large inward current that inactivates

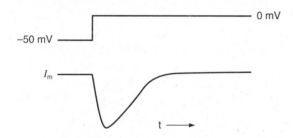

(c) Since nanananabooboolin appears to block the voltage-gated channels, these channels would not contribute to the current observed in the experiment. At a membrane potential of 0 mV one could expect almost complete activation of the voltage-gated Na⁺ channels, which would produce a large non-inactivating outward current.

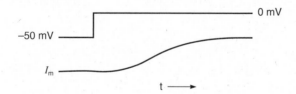

(d) The depolarization associated with the Cl⁻ action potential opens voltage-gated Ca²⁺ channels. Enough Ca²⁺ enters with this action potential to raise the intracellular concentration above the 1 µ*M* resting level, and this increase in concentration leads to the eversion of the spike-like spines.

8. (a) The minimum number of channels that can account for the records is two. During the step to +30 mV a number of unitary currents, each about 10 pA and each representing a single channel, are seen. There are also four events double the size of the unitary events. These double-sized events must represent two channels open simultaneously, i.e., there must be at least two channels in the patch recorded. The reason that such double-sized events are not seen at the lower step potentials is because the channels are voltage-gated; therefore the probability of each channel opening is low at these potentials and the probability of observing a double is low.

    (b) During the step to +30 mV the unitary currents through the voltage-gated K^+ channels are about 10 pA. Thus, the unitary conductance $\gamma_K = I_K/(V_m - E_K) = 83$ pS. During the step to –30 mV the unitary currents through the voltage-gated Na^+ channels are about 1.5 pA. Thus, the unitary conductance $\gamma_{Na} = I_{Na}/(V_m - E_{Na}) = 19$ pS. A unitary current of 1.5 pA means that 1.5 pC charge per second flows through the open voltage-gated Na^+ channels. Because there are 6.2×10^{18} charges per coulomb or 6.2×10^6 charges per pC, the flux through the open voltage-gated Na^+ channels recorded is 9.3×10^6 charges per second or about 10^7 charges per second as claimed in the textbook.

    (c) The electrochemical driving force $(V_m - E_{Na})$, moving K^+ outward, increases with increasing depolarization.

    The single-channel conductance γ_K of the open channel remains constant, regardless of the step potential.

    (d) Both the mean open time and the frequency of channel openings increase with increasing depolarization. These increases can be explained by the fact that the probability of channel opening increases with depolarization, i.e., the channels are voltage-gated.

    (e) The currents are inward for the Na^+ channel and outward for the K^+ channels at a step potential of –30 mV, because of the different electrochemical driving forces for the two ions at this potential $(V_m - E_{ion})$.

    The Na^+ channels inactivate during the voltage steps, while the K^+ channels do not. Thus, Na^+ channels open slowly at the beginning of the voltage steps, while K^+ channels continue to open throughout the duration of the voltage step.

    The K^+ channel openings occur with a greater lag after commencement of the voltage step than do the Na^+ openings, reflecting their slower activation kinetics.

(f) At a potential of –60 mV the voltage-gated K⁺ channels should have a very low probability of opening and open for a very brief time, i.e., activation is weak at this potential. The currents through the open channels should be small because the electrochemical driving force on K⁺ at this membrane potential ($V_m - E_K$) is small.

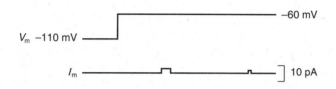

10. (a) $E_K = -80$ mV; $E_{Cl} = -60$ mV; $E_{Na} = +60$ mV.

(b) V_m (or E_m) = –65 mV.

(c) The late current represents outward current through voltage-gated K⁺ channels. With increasing depolarization the number of voltage-gated channels that open in response to the step in membrane potential increases. By about 0 mV all the available channels open, so the conductance increase to K⁺ is maximal at and above this potential. As the membrane potential steps increase, the electrochemical driving force moving K⁺ outward also increases, i.e., ($V_m - E_K$) becomes larger (more positive). Thus with increasing depolarization both increasing conductance and outward driving force work together to increase the late outward current, i.e., the K⁺ current.

The early current represents current through voltage-gated Na⁺ channels. The number of voltage-gated channel openings increases with depolarization. By about 0 mV all the available channels are open, so the conductance increase to Na⁺ is maximal at and above this potential. As the membrane potential steps increase, the electrochemical driving force moving Na⁺ inward *decreases,* i.e., $V_m - E_{Na}$ becomes smaller (less negative). At approximately +50 mV (i.e., at E_{Na}) the inward driving force becomes 0, and above this potential it becomes outward (i.e., $V_m - E_{Na}$ becomes positive). Thereafter, the driving force moving Na⁺ *outward* increases (becomes more positive) with increasing step potential. With increasing depolarization, conductance increases while inward driving force reverses and then becomes increasing but outwardly directed. Thus, with increasing depolarization the early current, i.e., the Na⁺ current, first increases due to the conductance increase in Na⁺, then decreases due to decreasing inward driving force, then reverses and increases due to increasing outward driving force.

(d)   The early current should be completely blocked and only a slowly activating late current should be measured.

(e)   Refer to Box 10–2 in the textbook to develop a strategy for calculating g_K. During the step to 0 mV the outward current is 2 μA. Thus, $g_K = I_K/(V_m - E_K) = 25$ μS.

(f)   This is very likely a voltage-gated K^+ channel. Since the current is outward at all the transpatch potentials tested and increases with increasing depolarization, K^+ is likely the permeant ion. The outward driving force on $K^+(V_m - E_K)$ should be positive at all the transpatch potentials tested and increase with increasing (more positive) V_m. The amount of time the channel spends in the open state increases with increasing depolarization, thus the channel is voltage-sensitive. The fact that openings are continuous throughout the trace indicates that the channel does not inactivate.

11

An Introduction to Synaptic Transmission

Overview

Synaptic transmission occurs at specialized junctions between neurons called synapses. Synapses may be either electrical or chemical. At electrical synapses the contact sites, called gap junctions, provide direct bridges between the cytoplasms of the pre- and postsynaptic neurons through which ions and small molecules pass. Thus transmission is by direct spread of ionic currents between neurons and is electrotonic and bidirectional. Electrical synapses are rapid and reliable, and they provide an efficient means of synchronous firing in groups of coupled neurons.

At chemical synapses the presynaptic terminal is specialized for the release of a chemical transmitter by exocytosis from intracellular vesicles. The postsynaptic cell is specialized to receive the chemical message via specific receptor proteins. These receptors can be of three types. An *ionotropic receptor* is itself an ion channel that is gated by the binding of the transmitter molecular. A *metabotropic receptor* is coupled via a G-protein to an ion channel or an enzyme that synthesizes intracellular second messenger(s). *Receptor tyrosine kinase* is an effector kinase. Transmission involving ionotropic receptors is said to be direct, while transmission involving metabotropic and receptor tyrosine kinase is indirect. Because several thousand transmitter molecules are released from each synaptic vesicle, there can be considerable amplification at chemical synapses.

Chemical synaptic transmission is quite plastic, being susceptible to a variety of modulatory and developmental influences; in particular, indirect transmission can serve to modulate direct transmission, leading to such phenomena as memory and learning. Electrical synaptic transmission can also be modulated by intracellular pH and Ca^{2+}, voltage, and phosphorylation by kinases, but is generally less plastic than chemical synaptic transmission.

Objectives

1. Understanding the similarities and differences between the two types of synaptic transmission, electrical and chemical.

2. Understanding the role of connexons in electrical synaptic transmission.

3. Understanding the similarities and differences between direct chemical synaptic transmission via ionotropic receptors and indirect chemical synaptic transmission via metabotropic or receptor tyrosine kinase.

4. Understanding the role of each type of synaptic transmission — electrical and direct and indirect chemical — in synaptic plasticity and putting each type into a behavioral context.

▰ *MATCHING PROBLEMS*

1. Distance between pre- and postsynaptic cell membranes at an electrical synapse or gap junction, in nm

   A. nearly 0

2. Distance between pre- and postsynaptic cell membranes at a chemical synapse, in nm

   B. 0.3 – 5

3. Typical distance between non-synaptic cell membranes in the nervous system, in nm

C. 1

4. Number of connexin protein subunits forming a connexon hemichannel

D. 1.5

5. Number of membrane-spanning regions in each connexin subunit

E. 2

6. Pore diameter of a gap junction channel when open, in nm

F. 3.5

7. Single-channel conductance of a gap junction channel when open, in pS

G. 4

8. Synaptic delay at an electrical synapse, in ms

H. 4

9. Synaptic delay at a chemical synapse, in ms

I. 5

10. Typical number of transmitter molecules in a synaptic vesicle

J. 6

11. Typical number of transmitter molecules that must bind to open an ionotropic receptor

K. 7

12. Typical number of protein subunits making up a ionotropic receptor

L. 20

13. Number of membrane-spanning regions for each subunit of an ionotropic receptor

M. 20 – 40

14. Number of protein subunits making up a metabotropic receptor

N. 100

15. Number of membrane-spanning regions for each subunit of a metabotropic receptor

O. several thousand

■ *TRUE/FALSE QUESTIONS*
(If false, explain why)

1. At electrical synapses gap junction channels provide direct bridges between the cytoplasm of pre- and postsynaptic neurons. _____

2. Transmission at electrical synapses is often called electrotonic because it is similar to passive spread of subthreshold electrical signals along axons. _____

3. Transmission at almost all electrical synapses is unidirectional. _____

4. Transmission at electrical synapses is seldom if ever modulated. _____

5. Intracellular Ca^{2+} concentration is thought to be a major modulator of gap junction channels. _____

6. The connexins from different tissues derive from several different gene families and share little structural similarity. _____

7. The cytoplasmic domains of connexin subunits of the gap junction channels vary greatly from tissue to tissue, and this variation may explain why gap junctions in different tissues are sensitive to different modulatory factors. _____

8. Electrical coupling among neurons by gap junctions lowers their collective threshold to excitatory synaptic input. _____

9. Electrical coupling among neurons by gap junctions leads to synchronous firing once threshold is exceeded. _____

10. At electrical synapses the presynaptic nerve terminal is usually much smaller than the postsynaptic neuron to increase the efficiency of transmission. _____

11. Electrical transmission is ideally suited for inhibition of postsynaptic neurons. _____

12. Small molecules other than ions do not pass between neurons coupled by gap junctions. _____

13. At chemical synapses the presynaptic nerve terminal can be much smaller than the postsynaptic neuron because the release of vesicles

containing several thousands of transmitter molecules amplifies the postsynaptic response. _____

14. At all chemical synapses there are specialized active zones in the presynaptic terminal. _____

15. Chemical synapses are unidirectional. _____

16. At chemical synapses the postsynaptic response is largely determined by the transmitter released and not by the type of postsynaptic receptor. _____

17. Chemical synapses require the influx of Ca^{2+} into the presynaptic terminal for the release of transmitter. _____

18. Metabotropic receptors are themselves ion channels. _____

19. Tyrosine kinase receptors and metabotropic receptors originate from different gene families. _____

20. G-proteins are so-called because they bind GTP. _____

21. G-proteins can activate enzymes that produce intracellular second messengers. _____

22. Chemical synapses are very rigidly fixed and show little synaptic plasticity compared to electrical synapses. _____

◼ SYNTHETIC QUESTIONS AND QUANTITATIVE PROBLEMS

1. Compare electrical synaptic transmission, chemical synaptic transmission involving ionotropic receptors, and chemical synaptic transmission involving metabotropic or tyrosine kinase receptors, with respect to speed, duration, and behavioral function.

2. It is often said that the differences between chemical synaptic transmission and endocrine function are blurry. Explain.

3. Delineate the steps in the process of chemical synaptic transmission from the arrival of the action potential at the presynaptic terminal to the postsynaptic response.

4. How does the humorous expression concerning human communication, "It's not what you say that matters, it's what ears your audience has on," apply to chemical synaptic transmission.

5. Use the computer program PSPSIM to explore how the size of an EPSP is related to the reversal potential of the EPSP, E_{EPSP}, the leakage conductance, g_l, and the conductance of the EPSP, g_{EPSP}. Set the simulation mode to Passive Membrane, EPSP, 1 Pulse. Vary the parameters using the option Post-Synaptic Parameters in the Mode menu. Use Measure to quantify your results. In each case observe the membrane currents associated with the EPSP by using Membrane Currents under the Plots menu. Push the Default button under Post-Synaptic Parameters if you make a mistake.

6. Use PSPSIM to explore synaptic integration. Use both Active and Passive Membrane under the Mode menu. Activate various combinations of EPSPs and EPSPs under Mode. Leave Post-Synaptic Parameters, Active Conductances, and Active $E_{(revs)}$ at default values. Observe the membrane currents associated with the EPSPs and EPSPs by using Membrane Currents under the Plots menu.

ANSWERS

■ MATCHING PROBLEMS

1. F.

2. M.

3. L.

4. J.

5. G.

6. D.

7. N.

8. A.

9. B.

10. O.

11. E.

12. I.

13. H.

14. C.

15. K.

■ TRUE/FALSE QUESTIONS

1. True

2. True

3. False. Transmission at almost all electrical synapses is *bi*directional.

4. False. Transmission at electrical synapses can *sometimes* be modulated.

5. True

6. False. The connexins from different tissues derive from *one* large gene family and share *considerable* structural similarity.

7. True

8. False. Electrical coupling among neurons by gap junctions *raises* their collective threshold to excitatory synaptic input.

9. True

10. False. At electrical synapses the presynaptic nerve terminal is usually much *larger* than the postsynaptic neuron to increase the efficiency of transmission.

11. False. Electrical transmission is ideally suited for *excitation* of post-synaptic neurons.

12. False. Small molecules other than ions *can often pass* between neurons coupled by gap junctions.

13. True

14. False. At *many but not all* chemical synapses there are specialized active zones in the presynaptic terminal.

15. True

16. False. At chemical synapses the postsynaptic response is largely deter-mined not by the transmitter released but by the type of postsynaptic receptor with which the transmitter interacts.

17. True

18. False. *Ionotropic* receptors are themselves ion channels.

19. True

20. True

21. True

22. False. Electrical synapses are relatively rigid and show little synaptic plasticity compared to chemical synapses.

SYNTHETIC QUESTIONS AND QUANTITATIVE PROBLEMS

1. Electrical transmission is very rapid and lasts only as long as the pre-synaptic neuron's electrical signal lasts. It is useful where faithful rapid transmission is needed, such as in neural networks that mediate escape behaviors, and in raising the collective threshold of a group of coupled neurons while ensuring that they fire together whenever threshold is reached.

   Chemical synaptic transmission involving ionotropic receptors can be relatively fast (as little as 0.3 ms synaptic delay), but it is slower than electrical transmission. The postsynaptic responses last only several milliseconds. Such chemical synapses are commonly found in neural circuits that directly mediate behavior.

   Chemical synaptic transmission involving metabotropic receptors or receptor tyrosine kinase is relatively slow and can last from several milliseconds to several seconds or minutes. Such synaptic actions often serve to modulate behavior by regulating the excitability and adjusting the strength of the ionophoric chemical synapses in the neural circuity mediating behavior.

2. Both chemical synaptic transmission and endocrine secretion involve the release of chemical signal molecules from vesicles by exocytosis. In general, however, hormones are released into the blood stream and transported to target tissues by the circulation, while neurotransmitters are released at synapses directly opposite postsynaptic receptors. This distinction is blurred by the fact that at some synapses, e.g., those at the smooth muscle of the gut, the presynaptic release sites are not closely associated with postsynaptic receptors, while some hormones are released locally and do not spread through the circulation. The same molecules can act as hormones, synaptic transmitters, and local messengers.

3. (a) The action potential arrives at the presynaptic terminal and provides depolarization that opens voltage-gated Ca^{2+} channels. (b) Calcium enters the presynaptic terminal, increasing the internal concentration of Ca^{2+}. (c) The increase in intracellular Ca^{2+} causes the exocytosis of vesicles containing a neurotransmitter. (d) The transmitter diffuses across the synaptic cleft and binds to postsynaptic receptors. (e) The postsynaptic receptors either directly gate ion channels (ionotropic receptors) or indirectly gate them and/or alter the metabolic processes of the postsynaptic neuron (metabotropic recep-

tors and receptor tyrosine kinase. (f) Synaptic transmission is terminated by diffusion of the transmitter from the synaptic cleft and destruction of the transmitter in the cleft by enzymes or reuptake of the transmitter into neurons or glia.

4. The postsynaptic receptor for a given transmitter, not the transmitter itself, determines the response to that transmitter. A given transmitter may act on a wide variety of receptors, including several types within each class — ionotropic, metabotropic, and tyrosine kinase — each coupled directly or indirectly to different ion channels or, in the case of metabotropic receptors and receptor tyrosine kinase, other intracellular effectors.

12

Transmission at the Nerve-Muscle Synapse

Overview

The vertebrate neuromuscular junction is characterized by a highly ordered structure known as the motor end-plate. When an action potential in a motor axon invades the presynaptic terminal at the end-plate, ACh is released from presynaptic vesicles at specialized active zones. The ACh diffuses across the synaptic cleft to nicotinic ACh receptors localized to the crests of junctional folds just opposite the active zones. These receptors are in fact ACh-activated ion channels, that, when open, allow cations such as Na^+ and K^+ to move through them. The opening of these ion channels causes a large depolarization of the postsynaptic membrane. Under normal conditions this depolarization is well above the threshold needed to trigger an action potential in the muscle fiber. The response to the released ACh is terminated when the ACh is destroyed by acetylcholinesterase in the basement membrane of the cleft or when the ACh diffuses away from the cleft.

The end-plate potential and its associated end-plate current can be studied better if its amplitude is reduced somewhat by curare, a competitive antagonist of nicotinic ACh receptors. When the postsynaptic fiber is voltage clamped, the end-plate current is found to have a reversal potential of approximately 0 mV. This observation is consistent with the idea that both Na^+ and K^+ flow through the open channel.

117

The activity of individual ACh-activated channels can be observed using the patch clamp technique. Each channel displays the same unitary conductance when activated by ACh. The size of the postsynaptic response to ACh is determined by the total number of ACh channels available, the probability that each channel is activated (determined by the concentration of ACh in the synaptic cleft), the single-channel conductance, and the electrochemical driving force at the postsynaptic membrane.

Each nicotinic ACh receptor-channel is made up of five protein subunits, two α units, and one each β, γ, and δ. Each subunit has four membrane-spanning regions, arranged such that the M2 region of each subunit forms the pore lining of the channel. There is a binding site for ACh on extracellular portions of each α subunit, and both these sites must be occupied by ACh for channel activation. Within the pore, three rings of negatively charged amino acids are thought to impart the cation selectivity to the channel.

Objectives

1. Understanding the structure of the vertebrate neuromuscular junction.

2. Understanding the postsynaptic mechanisms underlying the end-plate potential.

3. Understanding the relation between the end-plate potential and the end-plate currents as measured under voltage clamp.

4. Understanding the concept of reversal potential, especially as it applies to the end-plate current.

5. Understanding the structure and function of nicotinic ACh-activated channels and how their activity can account for the properties of the end-plate potential.

MATCHING PROBLEMS

1. Amplitude of the end-plate potential, in mV

    A. 0

2. Density of nicotinic ACh receptors at crests of the junctional folds, in receptors per μm^2

    B. 2

3. Width of the synaptic cleft, in nm

    C. 3

4. Single-channel conductance of the ACh-activated channel when open, in pS

    D. 4

5. Number of channel openings contributing to a normal end-plate current

    E. 4

6. Reversal potential of the end-plate current, in mV

    F. 5

7. Number of Na^+ ions that flow through an open ACh-activated channel at the resting potential

    G. 30

8. Number of subunits contributing to the ACh-activated channel

    H. 50

9. Number of ACh binding sites on the ACh-activated channel

    I. 70

10. Number of subunit types contributing to the ACh-activated channel

    J. 10,000

11. Number of membrane-spanning regions for each subunit of the ACh-activated channel

    K. 17,000

12. Number of negatively charged rings lining ACh-activated channel pore

    L. 200,000

■ TRUE/FALSE QUESTIONS
(If false, explain why)

1. The excitatory synaptic potential at the vertebrate neuromuscular junction is called the end-plate potential. _____

2. Every ACh-activated channel adds a different unitary conductance to the postsynaptic response. _____

3. The reversal potential of the end-plate potential and the single-channel currents through the ACh-activated channels at the neuromuscular junction are different because the ACh-activated channels rectify current. _____

4. The probability that an individual ACh-activated channel will open is independent of the concentration of ACh present. _____

5. The maximal size of the end-plate current is dependent on the total number of ACh-activated channels present at the neuromuscular junction. _____

6. The size of the end-plate current evoked by stimulation of the presynaptic motor neuron is independent of the potential at which the postsynaptic muscle fiber is held in voltage clamp. _____

7. The subunit structure of the nicotinic ACh-activated channel is $\alpha_2\beta\gamma\delta$. _____

8. The M3 membrane-spanning region of each subunit of the nicotinic ACh-activated channel forms the lining of the channel pore. _____

9. The positively charged amino acid lysine is the predominant one found in the three rings of charge of the pore lining in the nicotinic ACh-activated channel. _____

10. Both the amino and carboxyl termini of each subunit of the nicotinic ACh-activated channel are extracellular. _____

11. The fact that the duration of opening varies among individual channels in a population of ACh-activated channels can account for the fall-off of the end-plate current associated with an action potential in the presynaptic motor neuron. _____

12. The binding site for ACh is located on the γ subunit of the nicotinic ACh-activated channel. _____

SYNTHETIC QUESTIONS AND QUANTITATIVE PROBLEMS

1. Label the structures of the vertebrate neuromuscular junction in Figure 12–1 below.

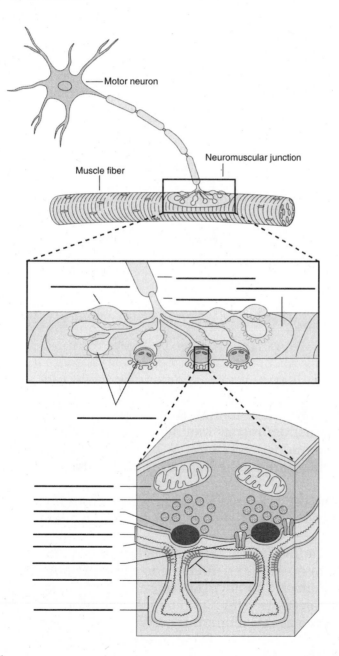

Figure 12–1

2. In the figure below draw in the correct total end-plate current and single-channel current in part A and indicate the magnitude and direction of each current or current component in part B, for each membrane potential.

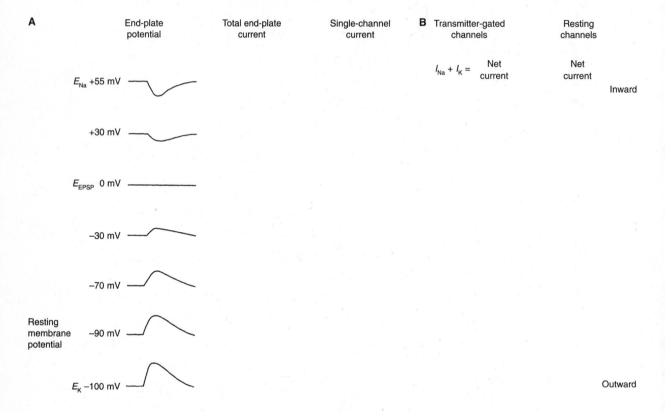

Figure 12–2

3. Define the reversal potential, E_{EPSP}, of the end-plate potential at the vertebrate neuromuscular junction in terms of the individual ionic currents that flow through the ACh-activated channels, and in terms of the equilibrium potentials of the ions involved.

4. How do the voltage-gated Na^+ channels of axons differ from the ACh-activated channels of the vertebrate neuromuscular junction?

5. Eserine is a drug that blocks the action of the enzyme acetylcholinesterase at the vertebrate neuromuscular junction. What effect would you predict eserine to have on the amplitude of the end-plate potential elicited by stimulation (depolarization) of the presynaptic motor neuron at this junction? Why?

6. A response very similar to the end-plate potential can be elicited at the vertebrate neuromuscular junction by brief direct focal application of ACh from a micropipette. What effects would eserine, curare, tetrodotoxin, and tetraethylammonium have on the response? Why?

7. Once again we return to the planet ZicZac, so refresh your memory of life here by referring to Quantitative Problems 8–4 (p. 67) and 10–7 (p. 93). Remember that when a polyseracyte feels the clammy pseudopod of a tyranocyte, it produces a Cl^- action potential that activates high-threshold voltage-gated Ca^{2+} channels. The resultant large Ca^{2+} influx causes a transient eversion of hundreds of spike-like spines that render it a bristly meal indeed. We never explored the mechanisms by which the membrane is brought to threshold for the generation of the Cl^- action potential (35 mV). You find that you can block the Cl^- action potential of the polyseracyte with a new drug nanananabooboolin, and under these conditions you find that the touch of the clammy pseudopod of a tyranocyte causes a maximum depolarization of 30 mV, which would be sufficiently large to reach threshold for a Cl^- action potential. This receptor potential is electrically equivalent to an excitatory synaptic potential like the end-plate potential at the vertebrate neuromuscular junction.

   The membrane of a polyseracyte contains ligand-gated channels that open when they bind a certain sugar residue attached to membranes of the clammy pseudopods of tyranocytes. These channels are extremely unusual because they allow both Cl^- and Na^+ to pass through them in a ratio of 1:2, and they account for the clammy pseudopod response (receptor potential) you observed.

   Expand the equivalent circuit diagram you drew for problem 8–4 to include these ligand-gated channels. What is the predicted reversal potential of the clammy pseudopod-mediated response, E_{cp}? What total conductance change, Δg_{cp}, brought about by the opening of the clammy pseudopod ligand-gated channels, would give rise to the observed maximal clammy pseudopod-mediated response?

ANSWERS

■ *MATCHING PROBLEMS*

1. I.

2. J.

3. H.

4. G.

5. L.

6. A.

7. K.

8. F.

9. B.

10. D.

11. E.

12. C.

■ *TRUE/FALSE QUESTIONS*

1. True

2. False. Every ACh-activated channel adds the *same* unitary conductance to the postsynaptic response.

3. False. The reversal potential of the end-plate potential and the single channels current through the ACh-activated channels at the neuromuscular junction are the *same*.

4. False. The probability that an individual ACh-activated channel will open is *dependent* on the concentration of ACh present.

5. True

6. False. The size of the end-plate current evoked by stimulation of the presynaptic motor neuron is *dependent* on the potential at which the postsynaptic muscle fiber is held in voltage clamp.

7. True

8. False. The *M2* membrane-spanning region of each subunit of the nicotinic ACh-activated channel forms part of the lining of the channel pore.

9. False. The negatively charged amino acids glutamate and aspartate are the predominant ones found in the three rings of charge of the pore lining in the nicotinic ACh-activated channel.

10. True

11. True

12. False. The binding site is located on the α subunit.

■ SYNTHETIC QUESTIONS AND QUANTITATIVE PROBLEMS

1. Check Figure 12–1 in the textbook (p. 198) for correct answers.

2. Check Figure 12–12 in the textbook (p. 208) for correct answers.

3. $V_m = E_{EPSP}$ when $I_K = I_{Na}$.

   $E_{EPSP} = (\Delta g_K E_K + \Delta g_{Na} E_{Na}) / (\Delta g_K + \Delta g_{Na})$.

4. ACh-activated channels are not voltage-gated, and they are not selective for Na⁺. Moreover, they are sensitive to a different array of drugs, e.g., α-bungarotoxin blocks the ACh-activated channels of the vertebrate neuromuscular junction, while tetrodotoxin blocks the voltage-gated Na⁺ channels of axons.

5. Eserine augments and prolongs the end-plate potential. Because eserine blocks acetylcholinesterase, more ACh makes it to the postsynaptic receptors and lasts longer in the synaptic cleft since only diffusion acts to remove it.

6. Eserine augments and prolongs the response to focal application of ACh. Because eserine blocks acetylcholinesterase, more ACh makes it to the postsynaptic receptors and it lasts longer in the synaptic cleft since only diffusion acts to remove it.
   Curare decreases, and can totally block, the response to focal application of ACh. Because curare binds to the ACh-activated channels and prevents ACh from binding, while not itself activating the channel, less activation of postsynaptic receptors occurs.

Tetrodotoxin and tetraethylammonium have no effect on the response to focal application of ACh. These drugs block voltage-gated Na$^+$ and K$^+$ channels respectively and have no effects on the ACh-activated channels that mediate the ACh response.

7. The electrical equivalent diagram below contains the ligand-gated channels.

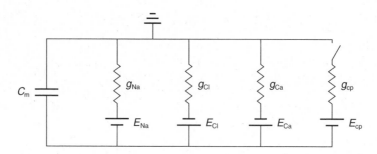

Refer to Box 12–1 in the textbook (p. 206) to develop the strategy for computing E_{cp}. You should obtain the following equation:

$$E_{cp} = \frac{\alpha E_{Cl} + E_{Na}}{\alpha + 1}$$

where:

$$\alpha = \frac{\Delta g_{Cl}}{\Delta g_{Na}} = 0.5$$

The correct answer is $E_{cp} = -19.3$ mV.

Refer to the postscript of Chapter 12 in the textbook (p. 213) to develop the strategy for computing the Δg_{cp} necessary for a maximal clammy pseudopod response, $\Delta V_{cp(max)}$, of 30 mV. Such a response means that the membrane potential at the peak of the response, $V_{cp(max)}$, will be 22 mV, since the resting potential, E_1, of a polyseracyte is 52 mV. You should obtain the following equation:

$$\Delta V_{cp(max)} \alpha = \frac{g_1 E_1 + \Delta g_{cp} E_{cp}}{g_1 + \Delta g_{cp}}$$

solving for Δg_{cp}, you obtain:

$$\Delta g_{cp} = \frac{g_1 \left(E_1 - V_{cp(max)} \right)}{V_{cp(max)} - E_{cp}}$$

The correct answer is $\Delta g_{cp} = 10.5 \times 10^{-6}$ S.

13

Synaptic Integration

Overview

The decision to fire an action potential is determined by the interaction of many (often tens to hundreds) excitatory and inhibitory synaptic inputs impinging onto a neuron. This decision, known as neuronal integration, is made at a specialized low-threshold trigger zone, where increased excitability is conferred by a high density of voltage-gated Na^+ channels. The trigger zone is often the axon hillock and is separate from the sites of inputs, dendrites, and cell bodies. Thus, the passive properties of neurons, particularly the length and time constants, play an important role in the integration of inhibitory and excitatory inputs, both spatially and temporally. (In neurons with extensive dendritic trees, specialized trigger zones in the dendrites employ voltage-gated Ca^{2+} channels to boost distant excitatory synaptic signals.)

The integration of inhibitory inputs is not simply a process of linear addition of EPSPs and IPSPs (EPSPs result from an increase in conductance of cations and a reversal potential usually around 0 mV, while IPSPs result from an increase in conductance of Cl^- and a reversal potential around –60 mV [E_{Cl}] or in some instances an increase in K^+ conductance with a reversal potential at E_K). The conductance change associated with IPSPs also shunts the effects of EPSPs and biases the membrane potential at the trigger zone toward the IPSP's reversal potential (–60 mV, or more negative, and thus well below threshold). The shape (geometry) of neurons and the placement of synaptic inputs thus play an important role in this synaptic

127

integration. Synaptic inputs onto axon terminals (axo-axonic synapses) serve mainly to modulate synaptic release and do not contribute to the neuron's decision to fire.

Synaptic excitation in the vertebrate central nervous system is mainly mediated by the neurotransmitter glutamate. Receptors for glutamate are both metabotropic and ionotropic. The ionotropic receptors are of two types, NMDA (named after the specific agonist N-methyl-D-aspartate) and non-NMDA. The non-NMDA receptor channels are selective for both K^+ and Na^+, but do not conduct Ca^{2+}. The NMDA receptor-channels, which conduct K^+, Na^+, and Ca^{2+}, are unique among transmitter-gated channels in that extracellular Mg^{2+} ions can block the channel at negative membrane potentials. Thus, NMDA channels require both glutamate and depolarization to open, i.e., they are voltage sensitive. This voltage sensitivity and the ability to conduct Ca^{2+}, which can activate Ca^{2+}/calmodulin-dependent protein kinase, gives them a role in synaptic plasticity.

Synaptic inhibition in the vertebrate central nervous system is mainly mediated by the neurotransmitter GABA and, to a lesser extent, glycine. GABA receptors are both ionotropic (GABA$_A$ conducting Cl^-) and metabotropic (GABA$_B$, leading to the opening of K^+ channels). Glycine receptors are ionotropic and conduct Cl^-.

Voltage-gated channels, transmitter-gated channels, and gap junction channels, although derived from different gene families, are structurally and functionally similar. Along with resting (leakage) channels, each plays a role in determining the electrical activity of neurons. Table 13–1 in the textbook (p. 240) highlights the contributions of these channels to the electrical signals observed in neurons, their mechanisms of action, and their ion selectivity.

Objectives

1. Understanding the basic mechanisms of neuronal integration: spatial summation, temporal summation and the integration of excitatory and inhibitor synaptic input.

2. Understanding excitatory and inhibitory synaptic mechanisms and the transmitters usually associated with these activities in vertebrates.

3. Understanding the unique properties of the NMDA receptor-channel that make possible its role in synaptic plasticity: voltage-sensitivity, the ability to conduct Ca^{2+}, and access to Ca^{2+}/calmodulin-dependent protein kinase.

4. Understanding the structural and functional similarities and differences among resting (leakage channels), voltage-gated channels, transmitter-gated channels, and gap-junction channels and their respective role in determining neuronal activity. Careful study of Table 13–1 in the textbook (p. 240) is recommended.

■ *MATCHING PROBLEMS*

1. Temporal summation

2. Initial segment of the axon or axon hillock

3. Decision to fire an action potential

4. Spatial summation

5. Dendritic trigger zones

6. Synaptic input zone representing a distinct biochemical compartment

7. Antagonist of NMDA receptors

8. Antagonist of non-NMDA receptors

9. Antagonist of metabotropic glutamate receptors

10. Natural ligand for NMDA and non-NMDA receptors

11. Agonists for non-NMDA receptors

12. Permeant ion(s) of non-NMDA receptor-channels

13. Permeant ions(s) of NMDA receptor-channels

14. Conductance of non-NMDA receptor-channels

A. CNQX

B. K^+, Na^+, and Ca^{2+}

C. voltage-dependent Ca^{2+} channels

D. < 20 ps

E. Cl^-

F. glutamate

G. Mg^{2+}

H. time constant

I. K^+ and Na^+

J. dendritic spine

K. low-threshold region, resulting from a high density of voltage-gated Na^+ channels

L. glycine

M. AMPA, kainate, and quisqualate

N. negatively charged flanking amino acids

15. Conductance of NMDA receptor-channels

    O. 10 nm cleft, small active zone, presynaptic projections less obvious, little or no basement membrane, oval or flattened vesicles (likely inhibitory)

16. Ion(s) which confer(s) voltage-sensitivity to NMDA receptor-channel

    P. 2-amino-5-phosphono-valeric acid (APV)

17. Necessary cofactor for functioning of the NMDA receptor-channel

    Q. ACPD

18. Permeant ion(s) of $GABA_A$ receptor channels

    R. 30 nm cleft, large active zone, dense presynaptic projections, round vesicles (likely excitatory)

19. Permeant ion(s) of $GABA_B$ receptor channels

    S. positively charged flanking amino acids

20. Permeant ion(s) of glycine receptor channels

    T. neuronal integration

21. Gray type I synapse

    U. Cl^-

22. Gray type II synapse

    V. 50 ps

23. M2 region of ACh receptor-channel

    W. length constant

24. M2 region of $GABA_A$ and glycine receptor-channels

    X. K^+

▪ *COMPLETION PROBLEMS*

1. The EPSP produced by one sensory sensory neuron on a spinal motor neuron depolarizes the motor neurons by less than _____, far below the threshold depolarization required for generating an action potential, which requires a depolarization of _____ or more.

2. As many as _____ to _____ presynaptic neurons must fire together to produce a synaptic potential large enough to trigger an action potential in a spinal motor neuron.

3. The net effect of the inputs at individual excitatory and inhibitory synapses depends on several factors: the _____, _____, and shape of the synapse, and the _____ and relative _____ of other synergistic or antagonistic synapses.

4. All three regions of a neuron — _____, _____, and _____ — can be receptive or transmitting sites for synaptic contact.

5. Synaptic current associated with the opening of ligand-gated channels always tends to drive the membrane potential toward the _____ of the synaptic currents, regardless of whether the initial membrane voltage is above or below the _____.

6. NMDA receptor channels are unique among ionotropic receptors in that external Mg^{2+} ions confer _____ on these channels.

▪ *TRUE/FALSE QUESTIONS*
(If false, explain why)

1. Dendritic trigger zones amplify weak excitatory input from remote parts of a dendrite. _____

2. Spatial summation is the process by which consecutive synaptic potentials at the same site are added together in the postsynaptic neuron. _____

3. Synaptic current generated at an axosomatic site has a weaker signal and thus less influence on the outcome at the trigger zone than does current from more remote axodendritic contacts. _____

4. In the brain, significant inhibitory input frequently occurs on the cell body of neurons because IPSPs generated here have a strong shunting effect on the trigger zone. _____

5. Synaptic inhibition is the result solely of the linear addition of IPSPs and EPSPs. _____

6. Ionotropic ACh receptors, GABA receptors, and glycine receptors arise from the same gene family. _____

7. The Ca^{2+} that enters through NMDA receptor-channels in the dendritic spines of CA1 pyramidal cells of the hippocampus can activate Ca^{2+}/calmodulin-dependent protein kinase. _____

8. The M2 region (the lining of the channel pore) of the nicotinic ACh receptor-channel is flanked by acidic amino acid residues such as glutamate and aspartate, while the M2 region of the glycine receptor-channel is flanked by basic amino acid residues such as lysine and arginine. _____

9. The $GABA_A$ receptor is metabotropic, while the $GABA_B$ receptor is ionotropic. _____

10. NMDA and non-NMDA channels are not related structurally and arise from only very distantly related gene families. _____

11. NMDA channels open and close very rapidly in response to glutamate. _____

12. Electrical current flow is always defined in terms of the flow of positive charge. _____

13. Synaptic inhibition is usually associated with the opening of Cl^- or K^+ channels. _____

14. GABA and glycine are generally thought of as excitatory transmitters in vertebrates. _____

15. The reversal potential for glutamate receptor-channel current is around 0 mV, while that of the $GABA_A$ channel current is around –60 mV. _____

16. The synaptic terminals of excitatory and inhibitory neurons can always be distinguished by their morphology. _____

17. The $GABA_A$ receptor is composed of at least three subunits: α, β, and γ. _____

18. PCP or "angel dust" is a noncompetitive antagonist of the NMDA receptor that acts by binding to a site in the open channel pore. _____

19. Two widely administered classes of drugs, benzodiazepines and barbiturates, both bind $GABA_A$ receptors and reduce the flux of Cl^- through these inhibitory channels in response to GABA. _____

20. Transmitter-gated, voltage-gated, and gap-junction channels are the products of different gene families and share little structural or functional similarity. _____

SYNTHETIC QUESTIONS AND QUANTITATIVE PROBLEMS

1. Demonstrate to yourself the shunting effect of inhibitory synaptic potentials by solving the following problem. Construct an equivalent circuit model of an area of dendritic membrane in which both excitatory and inhibitory receptor-channels coexist. Assume that the total resting conductance is 1 μS and that E_1 (or E_m, if you prefer) is –60 mV.

   (a) Calculate the peak size (in mV) of an EPSP mediated by both glutamate and non-NMDA receptors (assuming E_{EPSP} = 0 mV), if the associated conductance increase is 0.2 μS.

   (b) Calculate the peak (trough) size of an IPSP mediated by $GABA_A$ receptors (assuming E_{Cl} = –60 mV), if the associated conductance increase is 1.0 μS.

(c) Now assume that both synaptic potentials occur simultaneously; calculate the peak size (in mV) of the membrane depolarization.

2. Describe how you would determine experimentally the reversal potentials of an EPSP and IPSP.

3. How would you expect the records shown in Figure 13–11A in the textbook (p. 231) to differ if the experiment had been performed with no Mg^{2+} in the bathing medium?

4. Both nicotinic ACh receptor-channels and NMDA receptor-channels are permeable to cations (mainly Na+, K+, and Ca^{2+}) and both mediate EPSPs. In what significant way do these channels differ?

5. Voltage-gated channels are made up of polypeptides with four repeated segments with similar membrane-spanning motifs or domains. (Voltage-gated K^+ channels are composed of several, apparently four, subunits, each with a single similar membrane-spanning domain.) Transmitter-gated channels like the nicotinic ACh channel are composed of five subunits, each with a single similar membrane-spanning domain. Gap-junction channels are composed of six identical subunits, each with one membrane-spanning domain. What functional implications do the different numbers of membrane-spanning domains have for these three types of channels?

ANSWERS

■ MATCHING PROBLEMS

1.	H.	13.	B.
2.	K.	14.	D.
3.	T.	15.	V.
4.	W.	16.	G.
5.	C.	17.	L.
6.	J.	18.	E.
7.	P.	19.	X.
8.	A.	20.	U.
9.	Q.	21.	R.
10.	F.	22.	O.
11.	M.	23.	N.
12.	I.	24.	S.

■ *COMPLETION PROBLEMS*

1. 1 mV; 10 mV

2. 50–100

3. location; size; proximity; strength

4. axon; cell body; dendrites

5. reversal potential; reversal potential

6. voltage sensitivity

■ *TRUE/FALSE QUESTIONS*

1. True

2. False. *Temporal* summation is the process by which consecutive synaptic potentials at the same site are added together in the postsynaptic neuron.

3. False. Synaptic current generated at an axosomatic site has a *stronger* signal and thus *more* influence on the outcome at the trigger zone than does current from more remote axodendritic contacts.

4. True

5. False. Synaptic inhibition does not work solely by the linear addition of IPSPs to EPSPs, but also by clamping the membrane potential near the IPSP's reversal potential and by shunting EPSPs.

6. True

7. True

8. True

9. False. The GABA$_A$ receptor is ionotropic, while the GABA$_B$ receptor is metabotropic.

10. False. NMDA and non-NMDA channels *are related* structurallly and arise from a *single* gene family.

11. False. NMDA receptor-channels open and close very *slowly* in response to glutamate.

12. True

13. True

14. False. GABA and glycine are generally thought of as *inhibitory* transmitters in vertebrates.

15. True

16. False. The synaptic terminals of excitatory and inhibitory neurons can *sometimes* be distinguished by their morphology.

17. True

18. True

19. False. Two widely administered classes of drugs, benzodiazepines and barbiturates, both bind to GABA$_A$ receptors and *increase* the flux of Cl$^-$ through these inhibitory channels in response to GABA.

20. False. Transmitter-gated, voltage-gated, and gap-juction channels are the products of different gene families but have structural and functional similarities.

SYNTHETIC QUESTIONS AND QUANTITATIVE PROBLEMS

1. Refer to the postscript of Chapter 12 in the textbook (p. 213) and Quantitative Problem 12-7 (p. 126) to develop the strategy for computing the peak synaptic potential sizes.

   (a) 10 mV.

   (b) 0 mV. Because the reversal potential of the EPSP (i.e., E_{Cl}) is at the resting membrane potential (e.g., at rest Cl$^-$ is in equilibrium), the GABA-mediated increase in Cl$^-$ conductance does not produce a discernible synaptic potential at rest.

   (c) 5.5 mV. Although the GABA-mediated EPSP is not discernible at rest, it has a shunting effect that reduces the amplitude of the glutamate-mediated EPSP by nearly 50%.

2. Refer to Figures 13–8 and 13–12 in the textbook (p. 228, p. 233) to formulate your answer. Basically, both reversal potentials are determined in the same manner. Two electrodes in the postsynaptic cell, one for current injection (current clamp) and one for voltage recording, are used to set the membrane potential of the postsynaptic cell to a desired level. The PSP is then elicited by presynaptic stimulation and its amplitude and polarity are determined. In practice it is often difficult to determine the reversal potential of EPSPs by this method because the EPSPs reverse at relatively depolarized potentials; when the postsynaptic cell is brought to these potentials, action potentials and other conductance changes associated with the opening of voltage-gated channels by depolarization ensue. Thus, in practice it is often easier to determine the reversal potential of the excitatory postsynaptic current using voltage clamp. See Figure 13–8D in the textbook, p. 228.

3. With no Mg^{2+} in the bathing medium the NMDA receptor-channels will not be voltage sensitive; thus, they should open in response to glutamate regardless of the membrane potential at which the postsynaptic cell is held. The response in the presence of APV — the antagonist of NMDA receptors — will be identical, i.e., there will be no late current in the response. With no Mg^{2+} in the bathing medium, at a postsynaptic membrane potential of +20 mV the response without APV should be similar to that are shown in Figure 13–11 in the text-

book (p. 231), because at this potential in the presence of Mg^{2+} the NMDA receptor-channels can open normally in response to glutamate released by the presynaptic neuron. At a postsynaptic membrane potential of –80 mV, NMDA receptor-channels are nearly completely blocked by Mg^{2+}; at a membrane potential of –40 mV they are partially blocked by Mg^{2+}. Therefore, the responses without APV will be different, with and without Mg^{2+} in the bathing medium. In each case there should be considerably more late inward current, especially at the membrane potential of –80 mV, where the difference between Mg^{2+} and no-Mg^{2+} in blocking the NMDA receptors will be greatest.

4. Nicotinic ACh receptor-channels and NMDA receptor-channels differ in that Mg^{2+} in the extracellular medium confers voltage sensitivity to the NMDA receptor-channels — both the gating ligand (glutamate) and depolarization are necessary to open the NMDA receptor-channels. Such voltage sensitivity has not been observed for ACh receptor-channels.

5. Across these channel types a rough correlation is seen between channel pore size (and associated single-channel conductance) and the number of subunits or membrane-spanning domains. Thus, voltage-gated channels have the smallest pore size and single-channel conductance, while gap junction channels have the largest pore size and single-channel conductance. Transmitter-gated channels, like the nicotinic ACh channel, are intermediate.

14

Modulation of Synaptic Transmission: Second-Messenger Systems

Overview

Receptors that employ second messengers (metabotropic receptors) impart a tremendous flexibility and power to neurons and neural networks that is unattainable with ionophoric receptors. The use of second messengers prolongs the time scale of the response, amplifies the signal, and permits multiple points of control. The major second messengers include cAMP, DAG and PI_3, arachidonic acid, and its metabolites, cGMP, NO, and CO. Each of these second messengers is produced by a specific G-protein regulated enzyme. These stimulatory and inhibitory G-proteins are activated by metabotropic receptors when they bind their ligand.

Second-messenger systems can interact with one another through changes in internal Ca^{2+} concentration that arise from Ca^{2+} entry through voltage-gated channels or NMDA receptor-channels, and by release of Ca^{2+} from internal stores mediated by IP_3. Arguably, Ca^{2+} itself is a second messenger.

The effects of second-messenger systems on the electrical activity of neurons are mediated at several levels. Active G-proteins can directly open or close ion channels, second messengers themselves can open or close ion channels, or, most commonly, second messengers (sometimes in conjunction with Ca^{2+}) can activate protein kinases. These kinases phosphorylate channels or associated channel proteins, thereby opening or closing the channel or, in the case of voltage-gated channels, modifying its excitability. Protein kinases recognize specific amino acid sequences on target proteins, thus imparting specificity to second-messenger action and thus to receptor activation. In addition to ion channels, the targets of these kinases include other regulated proteins that affect other aspects of cellular metabolism and function. Moreover, second messengers, through their associated protein kinases, can directly regulate gene expression by activating (or inhibiting) response element-binding proteins.

Because second messengers can diffuse within a cell, they can affect all parts of the cell where they are generated, not just the subreceptor area. The arachidonic acid metabolites NO and CO are freely diffusible through cell membranes, and thus can leave the cell where they are produced and affect nearby cells. For this reason these molecules are often called transcellular messengers.

Postsynaptic responses mediated by second-messenger mediated responses are terminated by removal of the receptor ligand, hydrolysis of the activating GTP by the G-protein, destruction (or, for Ca^{2+}, internal sequestering) of the messenger molecule, and dephosphorylation of phosphorylated target proteins by protein phosphatases. Thus, the duration of second-messenger-mediated responses can be regulated at multiple levels and can be up to 10,000 times longer than responses mediated through ionotropic receptors.

Objectives

1. Understanding the major known second-messenger systems and their interactions.

2. Understanding how second-messenger systems amplify receptor activation and impart flexibility to neuronal function through their ability to both directly and indirectly modify channel function.

3. Understanding the role of G-proteins in mediating the effects of metabotropic receptors.

4. Understanding the role of protein kinases in mediating the effects of second messengers on channel activity and cellular metabolism.

5. Understanding the role of response element binding-proteins in mediating the effects of second messengers on gene transcription.

■ MATCHING QUESTIONS

1. Nicotinic ACh receptors, GABA$_A$ receptors, NMDA receptors

2. GABA$_B$ receptors, α- and β-adrenergic receptors

3. Growth factor receptors

4. Adenylyl cyclase

5. IP$_3$ and DAG

6. IP$_3$

7. Phospholipase A$_2$

8. Heme oxygenase

9. Nitric oxide synthetase

10. Ca^{2+}

11. DAG

12. Ca^{2+}/calmodulin-dependent protein kinase

13. Phospholipase C+ ADP

14. Arg-Arg-X-Ser-N.

15. Kinase regulatory subunit or domain

A. G-protein-coupled receptors

B. protein kinase C

C. requires an increase in internal Ca^{2+} concentration for activation

D. release of Ca^{2+} from internal stores

E. 12-lipoxygenase, 5-lipoxygenase, and cyclooxygenase

F. pseudosubstrate

G. cyclooxygenase

H. phosphatidylinositol (PI)

I. CO

J. protein + ATP $\rightarrow$ protein-P + ADP

K. ligand-gated ion channels

L. receptor tyrosine kinase

M. arachidonic acid

N. phosphorylation sequence

O. ATP $\rightarrow$ cAMP + PP$_i$

16. Eicosanoid metabolites of arachidonic acid

17. Prostaglandins and thromboxanes

18. Transcellular messengers

19. Tyrosine kinases

20. Phosphodiesterase

21. Protein phosphatases

22. Cholera toxin

23. Pertussis toxin

24. Phorbol esters

25. Protein kinase

26. Possible retrograde synaptic messengers

P. G_i or G_o

Q. NO

R. eicosanoids, NO, and CO

S. calmodulin

T. G_s

U. eicosanoids, NO, and CO

V. activators of protein kinase C

W. cAMP → AMP

X. protein P → protein + P_i

Y. PI → IP_3 and DAG

Z. autophosphorylation

COMPLETION PROBLEMS

1. The S-type K^+ channel of the marine snail *Aplysia* is closed by serotonin with _____ acting as the second messenger, and is opened by the peptide Phe-Met-Arg-Phe-NH$_2$ with _____ acting as the second messenger.

2. Closing of the S-type K^+ channel of the marine snail *Aplysia* by serotonin is associated with _____ of the channel or a channel regulatory protein, while opening of this channel by Phe-Met-Arg-Phe-NH$_2$ is associated with _____ of the second messenger.

3. Synaptic actions mediated by second messengers last up to _____ longer than directly mediated actions through ionotropic receptors.

4. Neurotransmitters can increase the internal Ca^{2+} concentration of cells through three different pathways: (1) _____ from internal stores by _____, (2) entry through _____ Ca^{2+} channels on the surface membrane when the membrane potential is depolarized by a transmitter, and (3) entry through _____ receptors on the surface membrane.

5. Receptor desensitization has been associated with _____.

6. The second messenger cAMP can influence gene expression by causing _____ to be phosphorylated by cAMP-dependent protein kinase.

▇ *TRUE/FALSE QUESTIONS*
(If false, explain why)

1. The functional diversity among different G-proteins derives mainly from differences in the α subunits rather than in the β or γ subunits. _____

2. All G-protein-coupled receptors discovered to date have seven membrane-spanning regions. _____

3. Once a G-protein is activated by interacting with an active receptor (with its ligand bound), it must act through a second-messenger producing enzyme before it can influence channel activity. _____

4. Phosphorylation rarely if ever induces a conformational change in the phosphorylated protein. _____

5. Regulated proteins, e.g., enzymes, often contain several different potential phosphorylation sites, which are the substrates for different specific protein kinases. _____

6. The second messenger IP_3, which is produced from the membrane phospholipid PIP_2, is restricted to the membrane after it is produced because it is not soluble in the cytoplasm (water). _____

7. The endoplasmic reticulum acts as a reservoir of Ca^{2+}, which can be released into the cytoplasm by IP_3. _____

8. Carbon monoxide is a deadly poison and thus cannot be used as a transcellular second messenger. _____

9. Nitric oxide is the same as the laughing gas used by dentists for anesthesia. _____

10. The M-type K^+ channel is a voltage-dependent channel that can be closed by activation of muscarinic ACh receptors. _____

11. Once they are activated, receptor tyrosine kinases usually act as dimers by binding their ligand. _____

12. Activation of a G-protein is associated with the hydrolysis of a bound GTP to GDP + P_i. _____

13. Voltage-gated ion channels can be modulated through the action of metabotropic receptors. _____

14. Second messengers and G-proteins can act directly on ion channels. _____

15. By opening K^+ channels, norepinephrine increases excitability and overrides spike accommodation in hippocampal neurons. _____

16. Response element-binding proteins are *cis*-acting elements regulating gene expression. _____

17. An enhancer is a *trans*-acting element regulating gene expression. _____

18. A TATA box is a common component of the promoter region of a gene. _____

■ SYNTHETIC QUESTIONS AND QUANTITATIVE PROBLEMS

1. Complete the figure below by filling in appropriate terms in each empty box.

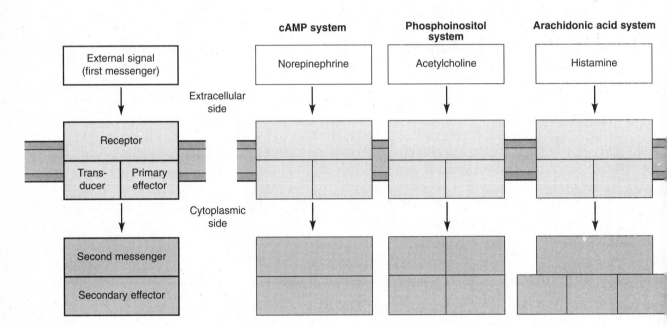

Figure 14–1

2. Assume that a slow EPSP, like that mediated by LHRH in sympathetic ganglia (see Figure 14–12 in the textbook, p. 259), is produced through the cAMP second-messenger pathway and involves the G-protein G_s. Assume further that the postsynaptic cells that show this response are easily accessible for intracellular recording, stimulation, and microinjection.

   (a) IBMX, a methylxanthine, can block the activity of phosphodiesterase, the enzyme that destroys cAMP, by converting it to AMP. What effect would you expect IBMX to have on this slow EPSP?

   (b) Cholera toxin can ADP-ribosylate G_s and render it unable to hydrolyze GTP. What effect would you expect cholera toxin to have on this slow EPSP?

   (c) What effect would intracellular injection of the catalytic subunit of cAMP-dependent protein kinase have on the postsynaptic cells?

(d) You have available a molecularly engineered form of the regulatory subunit of cAMP-dependent protein kinase, one that lacks a cAMP binding site but retains its ability to bind with other regulatory subunits and the catalytic subunits. What effect would intracellular injection of this subunit have on the slow EPSP?

3. Fill in the table below.

	Ion Channels Involved	*Effect on Total Membrane Conductance*	*Contributions to Action Potential*	*Time Course*	*Second Messenger*	*Nature of Synaptic Action*
EPSP due to opening of ion channels						
EPSP due to closing of ion channels						

4. In chronically stressed animals, adrenergic neurons increase their neuronal levels of norepinephrine. Discuss the mechanisms by which this stress-induced increase may occur.

5. Convince yourself that decreased-conductance EPSPs, like that mediated by LHRH in sympathetic ganglia (see Figure 14–12 in the textbook), actually augment the action of increased-conductance EPSPs, by solving the following problem using an equivalent circuit model of an area of dendritic membrane. Assume a nonmodifiable resting conductance of 1 μS and a leakage reversal potential of –60 mV, i.e., in the equivalent circuit $G_1 = 1.0$ μS and E_1 (or E_m, if you prefer) = –60 mV. Assume that in parallel with the nonmodifiable leakage channels are K^+ leakage-like channels with a total conductance of 0.5 μS, which close when phosphorylated in response to LHRH. Assume that E_K is –70 mV.

(a) Calculate the apparent resting potential of the cell.

(b) Calculate the peak size (in mV) of an EPSP mediated by LHRH if all the leak-like K^+ channels are closed.

(c) Calculate the peak size of an EPSP mediated by ACh through nicotinic receptors (assume $E_{EPSP} = 0$ mV) if the associated conductance increase is 0.2 μS.

(d) Now assume that both synaptic potentials occur simultaneously.

Calculate the peak size (in mV) of the ACh-mediated EPSP and the total membrane depolarization.

6. Discuss ways in which the electrophysiological effects mediated by metabotropic receptors differ from those mediated by ionotropic receptors.

ANSWERS

MATCHING PROBLEMS

1. K.

2. A.

3. L.

4. O.

5. H.

6. D.

7. M.

8. I.

9. Q.

10. S.

11. B.

12. C.

13. Y.

14. N.

15. F.

16. E.

17. G.

18. R.

19. Z.

20. W.

21. X.

22. T.

23. P.

24. V.

25. J.

26. U.

COMPLETION PROBLEMS

1. cAMP; arachidonic acid

2. phosphorylation; direct action

3. 10,000 times

4. release; IP_3; voltage-gated; NMDA

5. protein phosphorylation

6. CREB

TRUE-FALSE QUESTIONS

1. True

2. True

3. False. Once a G-protein is activated by interacting with an active receptor (with its ligand bound), it can act through a second-messenger producing enzyme or in some cases can interact directly with an ion channel to influence channel activity.

4. False. Phosphorylation *usually* induces a conformational change in the phosphorylated protein.

5. True

6. False. The second messenger IP_3, which is produced from the membrane phospholipid PIP_2, *is soluble* in water and freely diffuses through the cytoplasm after it is produced.

7. True

8. False. Although carbon monoxide is a deadly poison, it *is* used as a transcellular second messenger.

9. False. Nitric oxide, NO, is different from laughing gas (nitrous oxide, N_2O) used by dentists for anesthesia.

10. True

11. True

12. False. During activation of a G-protein, bound GDP is displaced by GTP.

13. True

14. True

15. False. By *closing* K^+ channels, norepinepherine increases excitability and overrides spike accomodation in hippocampal neurons.

16. False. Response elements (enhancers) are the targets of response element-binding proteins and are *cis*-acting elements regulating gene expression.

17. False. An enhancer is a *cis*-acting element regulating gene expression.

18. True

◼ *SYNTHETIC QUESTIONS AND QUANTITATIVE PROBLEMS*

1. See Figure 14–2 in the textbook, p. 245.

2. (a) IBMX should prolong and even enhance the slow EPSP because, by preventing the breakdown of cAMP, higher levels of cAMP will accumulate and persist for a longer time. Thus, the activation of cAMP-dependent protein kinase will be enhanced and prolonged; therefore, the closure of K^+ channels associated with the slow EPSP will be enhanced and prolonged.

(b)   Cholera toxin should prolong and even enhance the slow EPSP, because it prevents deactivation of G_s once it is activated by a ligand-bound receptor and itself binds a GTP. Until the bound GTP is hydrolyzed, which is prevented by ADP-ribosylation, G_s will remain active and can then activate adenylyl cyclase. Thus, higher levels of cAMP will be produced and accumulate over a longer time, the activation of cAMP-dependent protein kinase will be enhanced and prolonged, and the closure of K^+ channels associated with the slow EPSP will be enhanced and prolonged.

(c)   Intracellular injection of the catalytic subunit of cAMP-dependent protein kinase would produce a persistent depolarization through prolonged closure of K^+ channels associated with the slow EPSP. Only after the cell was able to neutralize the effects of the catalytic subunits of cAMP-dependent protein kinase with excess regulatory subunits would the depolarization subside.

(d)   If enough of the mutant subunit kinases were injected, the cell would no longer be responsive to LHRH because increases in intracellular cAMP levels associated with LHRH receptor activation could not relieve the blockade of the catalytic subunits of cAMP-dependent protein kinase by the mutant regulatory subunits. Smaller amounts of injected regulatory subunits would partially block the LHRH-mediated EPSP.

3.   See Table 14–1 in the textbook, p. 259.

4.   Stress, through increased cholinergic presynaptic input, causes increased release of norepinephrine. Activation of metabotropic ACh receptors on the adrenergic neurons and the subsequent rise in intracellular cAMP can compensate for the increased norepinephrine release by two basic mechanisms. (1) cAMP-dependent protein kinase phosphorylates tyrosine hydroxylase (the enzyme that catalyzes the rate-limiting step in norepinephrine biosynthesis) and relieves it of end product inhibition, so that it is more active and more norepinephrine is produced. (2) persistent stress leads to persistent large increases in cAMP, so that enough cAMP-dependent protein kinase is activated to lead to the phosphorylation of the cAMP-response-element binding protein (CREB) that activates transcription of the tyrosine hydroxylase gene. Consequently, more of this enzyme is made. The increase in tyrosine hydroxylase activity leads to lasting increases in norepinephrine production.

5.   Refer to the postscript of Chapter 12 in the textbook (p. 213) and Quantitative Problem 12–7 (p. 123) to develop a strategy for answering this question. Also, compare your results with those from

Quantitative Problem 13–1 (p. 138) where you demonstrated the shunting effect of an increased conductance IPSP.

(a) To calculate the apparent resting potential, treat the modifiable leakage-like K^+ channels as parallel open K^+ channels, $g_{K(LHRH)}$.

$$V_m = [g_l(E_l) + g_{K(LHRH)}(E_K)]/[g_l + g_{K(LHRH)}] = -63 \text{ mV} = E_{m(apparent)}$$

(b) The peak size of the LHRH-mediated EPSP, if all the modifiable leakage-like K^+ channels are closed, will be 3 mV because the membrane potential will return to $E_l = -60$ mV.

(c) Treat the modifiable leakage-like K^+ channels as leakage, thus:

$$g_{l(apparent)} = [g_l + g_{K(LHRH)}] = 1.5 \text{ } \mu S.$$

$$E_{m(apparent)} = -63 \text{ mV.}$$

$$V_{EPSP(ACh)} =$$

$$[G_{l(apparent)}(E_{m(apparent)}) + g_{EPSP(ACh)} E_{EPSP(ACh)}] /$$
$$[G_{l(apparent)} + g_{EPSP(ACh)}] = -56 \text{ mV}$$

(d) The LHRH-mediated EPSP will cause the membrane potential to return to $E_l = -60$ mV. At this potential

$$V_{EPSP(ACh)} = [g_l(E_l) + g_{EPSP(ACh)} (E_{EPSP(ACh)})] / [g_l + g_{EPSP(ACh)}] = -50 \text{ mV.}$$

The membrane will be depolarized to –50 mV and the size of the ACh mediated EPSP will be [–50 (–60)] = 10 mV. Hence, the LHRH-mediated EPSP augments the ACh-mediated EPSP by 1 mV.

6. Ionotropic receptors are receptor-channels that are gated open when their specific gating ligand is bound. The conductance increase, associated with the opening of the ion channels, produces the effects of ionotropic receptors on the electrical activity of neurons. In general, the ionotropic receptor-channels are not voltage-sensitive and do not flux Ca^{2+} ions. An important exception to these two generalizations is the NMDA receptor-channel, which is voltage-sensitive; it requires depolarization to relieve blockade of the channel by extracellular Mg^{2+} and fluxes Ca^{2+}. These special characteristics endow the NMDA receptor with special functional properties that make it important in synaptic plasticity. Because the effects on ion channels are direct, they are rapid in onset and last only as long as the gating ligand is present. The effects of ionotropic receptors are localized to the area of the membrane where the receptors are activated.

    Metabotropic receptors act through G-proteins and indirectly affect ion channels to exert their effects on the electrical activity of neurons.

The G-proteins can interact directly with ion channels or, more commonly, with enzymes that produce (or in some cases destroy) intracellular second messengers. These second messengers can then interact directly with ion channels or, more commonly, they activate protein kinases that act on channels, by phosphorylating these channels or channel associated proteins. Because they work through intracellular molecules — G-proteins, second messengers, protein kinases, and phosphorylated channels — that are relatively slow to activate and build up and are often persistent, the effects of metabotropic receptors are slower to develop and can be quite long-lasting. The channels that are modified can be either gated open or gated closed; thus both increases and decreases in conductances are possible. Moreover, the modulated channels can be voltage-gated channels that either contribute to the excitability of neurons (K^+ channels, for example) or participate in regenerative potentials like the action potential (e.g., voltage-gated Na^+ or Ca^{2+} channels). Because the second messengers and activated kinases are often diffusible, metabotropic receptors can exert effects on ion channels throughout a neuron.

15

Transmitter Release

Overview

Synaptic transmission provides the functional linkage between neurons that makes possible modifiable neural networks that can program, control, and modulate behavior.

Voltage-gated Ca^{2+} channels, which occur in relatively high density in presynaptic terminals, convert the electrical signals used for high-speed transmission along the axon into secretory signals that can pass from one neuron to the next. The influx of Ca^{2+} through these channels influences the release of synaptic vesicles filled with transmitter in two ways. Calcium triggers vesicle fusion, leading to transmitter release by exocytosis when a vesicle is docked at an active zone, probably by causing dilation in a fusion pore that traverses both the vesicle and plasma membrane. Calcium also regulates the targeted transport of vesicles to the active zone by freeing vesicles from their cytoskeletal tethers through the action of Ca^{2+}/calmodulin-dependent protein phosphorylation.

We are now only beginning to understand the molecular mechanisms involved in calcium-triggered synaptic transmission. Each step in the process has been delineated, and proteins thought to be involved in each one have been identified. The steps include: the filling of synaptic vesicles with transmitter, the tethering of synaptic vesicles to the cytoskeleton, the freeing of vesicles from their cytoskeletal tethers, the targeting of freed vesicles to the active zone, the docking of the vesicles at the active zone in preparation for release, the formation and opening of the fusion pore for release, and vesicle recycling.

Because synaptic transmission involves exocytosis of a uniform population of transmitter vesicles, synaptic transmission is necessarily quantized. Statistical analysis of the size variation of synaptic potentials is consistent with the notion of independent quantal release of transmitter, and morphological studies at the ultrastructural level confirm the vesicle hypothesis. In some cells, as in the retina, synaptic transmission may not involve exocytosis from vesicles but may be accomplished by reversal of transmitter transporters.

Extrinsic or intrinsic factors can modify transmitter release by influencing the influx of Ca^{2+} or modifying the release machinery itself. Because of the dual role calcium plays in vesicle fusion and mobilization, modulation of Ca^{2+} influx is a particularly important means of influencing transmitter release. In many neurons presynaptic inhibition and facilitation are produced by mechanisms that alter Ca^{2+} influx, for example through modulation of presynaptic voltage-gated Ca^{2+} or K^+ channels. Likewise, posttetanic potentiation may be produced through increased vesicle mobilization caused by the buildup of residual Ca^{2+} following tetanic activity.

Long-term changes in synaptic strength are probably due to growth or retraction of synaptic terminals rather than just modification of Ca^{2+} influx (or modulation of the release machinery), but Ca^{2+} influx may play a role in bringing about these changes.

Objectives

1. Understanding the role of presynaptic voltage-gated Ca^{2+} channels and Ca^{2+} influx in synaptic transmission.

2. Understanding the quantal nature of synaptic transmission.

3. Understanding the role of synaptic vesicles in synaptic transmission.

4. Understanding the outlines of the molecular machinery involved in vesicle tethering, mobilization and targeting to the active zone, docking at the active zone, opening of the fusion pore, and recycling and refilling.

5. Understanding how extrinsic and intrinsic factors regulate transmitter release by influencing Ca^{2+} influx in the presynaptic cell and modification of the release machinery.

▪ COMPLETION PROBLEMS

1. At the vertebrate neuromuscular junction the elementary ACh potential produced by the opening of a single channel is only about 0.3 μV, or about 1/200,000th of the amplitude of the _____.

2. At the vertebrate neuromuscular junction, in the presence of elevated external Mg^{2+} and reduced external Ca^{2+}, it is possible to record a unit synaptic potential in response to an action potential that is identical in _____ and _____ to the _____.

3. At the vertebrate neuromuscular junction alterations in the external Ca^{2+} concentration do not effect the _____ of a quantum, but rather the _____ that a quantum will be released.

4. The large quantal content (average number of vesicles released by a presynaptic action potential) of the vertebrate neuromuscular junction is associated with a large presynaptic area (_____ to _____ $μM^2$) in which about _____ active zones are distributed with about _____ associated vesicles.

5. At the vertebrate neuromuscular junction all end-plate potentials larger than the unit synaptic potential are _____ of the unit potential.

6. At the vertebrate neuromuscular junction the large intramembranous particles observed (using the freeze-fracture technique) along the dense bar or active zone are thought to be _____.

7. Calcium contributes to two aspects of vesicle function during synaptic transmission: _____ of synaptic vesicles from the storage pool attached to the cytoskeleton and dilation of the _____.

8. The transient fusion pore generated during exocytosis of transmitter from a vesicle has a diameter of _____ nm and a conductance of _____ pS.

9. During normal activity at the frog neuromuscular junction the predominant pathway for vesicle recycling involves endocytosis of _____.

10. The most likely mechanism for posttetanic potentiation is the buildup of residual _____, which causes increased _____ of synaptic vesicles for release.

11. Because axo-axonic synapses can control the _____ into synaptic terminals, they can depress or enhance _____ .

■ *TRUE/FALSE QUESTIONS*
(If false, explain why)

1. When voltage-gated Na^+ and K^+ channels are blocked with TTX and TEA respectively, synaptic transmission at the squid giant synapse is smoothly graded with presynaptic depolarization up to a saturating plateau level. _____

2. Presynaptic voltage-gated Ca^{2+} channels at the squid giant synapse inactivate quickly upon depolarization. _____

3. Calcium entry through voltage-gated Ca^{2+} channels during a presynaptic action potential can increase the Ca^{2+} concentration at the active zone a thousandfold within a few hundred microseconds. _____

4. The small time necessary to increase the Ca^{2+} concentration in the presynaptic terminal during an action potential to reach levels that cause synaptic release does not contribute significantly to the synaptic delay. _____

5. The Ca^{2+} current responsible for transmitter release at the squid giant synapse is smoothly graded in proportion to the level of depolarization of the presynaptic cell. _____

6. The duration of an action potential is an important determinant of the amount of Ca^{2+} that flows into a presynaptic terminal and hence of the amount of transmitter released. _____

7. Calcium influx through N- and P-type Ca^{2+} channels contributes directly to transmitter release in many vertebrate neurons. _____

8. At the vertebrate neuromuscular junction the unit synaptic potential, representing the release of a single quantum of transmitter, cannot be equated with the spontaneous miniature end-plate potential. _____

9. About 5,000 molecules of ACh are needed at the vertebrate neuromuscular junction to produce one miniature end-plate potential. _____

10. Miniature end-plate potentials are unaffected by the cholinergic drugs prostigmine or curare. _____

11. At the vertebrate neuromuscular junction, in the presence of elevated external Mg^{2+} and reduced external Ca^{2+}, increasing the external Ca^{2+} concentration increases the size of the unit synaptic potential. _____

12. The Ca^{2+} that enters the presynaptic terminal at the vertebrate neuromuscular junction during an action potential transiently increases the rate of quantal release 100,000-fold, bringing about the synchronous release of 150 quanta of transmitter (ACh). _____

13. At the vertebrate neuromuscular junction and the squid giant synapse the number of vesicles (quanta) released by a presynaptic action potential is between 100 and 300, but at most central synapses of vertebrates the number of vesicles (quanta) released by the action potential is between 1 and 10. _____

14. A miniature end-plate potential of 0.5 mV represents the opening of 2,000 ACh receptor-channels. _____

15. The exocytosis of transmitter from vesicles decreases the electrical capacitance of secretory cells. _____

16. Transmitter release at all chemical synapses is accomplished by exocytosis from vesicles. _____

17. Morphological studies at the vertebrate neuromuscular junction provide independent evidence that synaptic vesicles store transmitter and that exocytosis is the mechanism by which transmitter is released into the synaptic cleft. _____

18. Transmitter release can be accomplished by reversal of transporter proteins. _____

19. Just outside the active zone a reserve pool of transmitter-filled vesicles is held anchored to actin filaments of the cytoskeleton. _____

20. Freeing of vesicles tethered to the cytoskeleton in the storage pool is brought about by phosphorylation of synapsin by Ca^{2+}/calmodulin-dependent protein kinase. _____

21. Synaptotagmin is a calcium-binding protein involved in the docking and fusion of synaptic vesicles. _____

22. Rab 3 proteins are ATP-binding proteins that assist in vesicle docking. _____

23. Modulation of voltage-gated K^+ channels in presynaptic terminals can regulate Ca^{2+} influx and thus transmitter release. _____

24. Increased Cl^- conductance in presynaptic terminals can augment the amplitude of the action potential and thus cause presynaptic facilitation. _____

25. The release machinery itself is not modulated by presynaptic neural input to regulate transmitter release. _____

26. Direct modulation of presynaptic voltage-gated Ca^{2+} channels is an effective way of regulating transmitter release. _____

27. Modulation of action potential duration is not an effective way to regulate transmitter release. _____

SYNTHETIC QUESTIONS AND QUANTITATIVE PROBLEMS

1. Fill in the missing labels of the two schematic views of the neuromuscular junction.

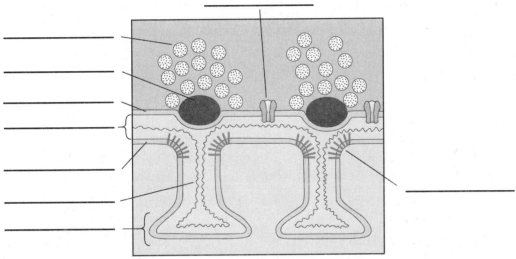

A. Cross section as in conventional transmission electron microscopy.

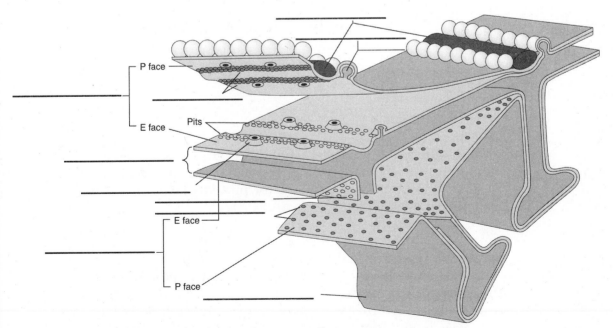

B. Three-dimensional view as in freeze fracture electron microscopy.

Figure 15–1

2. (a) Specific proteins and classes of proteins are thought to be involved in the *filling* of synaptic vesicles with transmitter, the *tethering* of synaptic vesicles to the cytoskeleton, the *freeing* of vesicles from their cytoskeletal tethers, the *targeting* of freed vesicles to the active zone, the *docking complex* for the vesicles in preparation for release, the formation and dilation of the *fusion pore* for release, and vesicle *recycling*. Identify the putative function of each protein (or protein class) in the following list.

Calcium/calmodulin-dependent protein kinase

Clathrin

Neurexins

NSF

Physophillin

Rab proteins

α-SNAP, γ-SNAP, SNAP-25

Synapsins

Synaptophysin

Syntaxins

VAMPs (synaptobrevin)

Vesicle transporters

(b) The toxins botulinum toxin, tetanus toxin, and α-latrotoxin are thought to exert their effects on synaptic transmission by interacting with one of the proteins (or protein classes) listed in (a). Identify the target for each toxin.

3. Assume that you can make an experimental preparation of the squid giant synapse like that used to generate the data in Figures 15–1 and 15–3 in the textbook (p. 270, p. 273), and that you perform all of the electrophysiological measurements and manipulations illustrated in those figures. Assume that you know that the transmitter used by this synapse is ACh, and that the postsynaptic ACh receptors are nicotinic and can be blocked by curare (this assumption is incorrect, as glutamate is the probable transmitter, but the logic of the question is not

influenced by this fact). Assume that you can focally apply ACh from a micropipette directly onto the postsynaptic membrane and evoke a depolarizing response similar to the EPSP, henceforth called the ACh response. Assume that replacement of Ca^{2+} ions in the bathing medium with Co^{2+} ions will effectively block voltage-gated Ca^{2+} channels. Assume that you are able to microinject drugs and polypeptides into the presynaptic terminal at will.

You apply TTX and TEA to the preparation and depolarize the presynaptic terminals with injected current as illustrated in Figure 12–2 in the textbook (p. 272). Under these conditions you are able to record an EPSP evoked by the presynaptic depolarization that is graded in proportion to the level of the depolarization and an ACh response that is graded in proportion to the amount of ACh applied.

(a)   What effect will replacing Ca^{2+} ions with Co^{2+} ions in the bathing medium have on the EPSP and the ACh response? Why?

(b)   What effect will injection of the presynaptic terminal with botulinum toxin have on the EPSP and the ACh response? Why?

(c)   What effect will adding prostigmine (an acetylcholinesterase inhibitor) and curare to the bathing medium have on the EPSP and the ACh response? Why?

(d)   What effect will replacing half of the Na^+ in the bathing medium with an impermeant ion have on the EPSP and the ACh response? Why?

(e)   A new toxin extracted from the venom of the New York sewer spider, kandelotoxin, when added to the bathing medium blocks the EPSP but not the ACh response. Propose a site of action for kandelotoxin and justify your answer.

(f)   You step the presynaptic potential from –80 mV to 0 mV and back, and record the Ca^{2+} current and postsynaptic potential illustrated in A below. Note that the Ca^{2+} current does not inactivate during the voltage step and turns off (deactivates) slowly after the step. The synaptic potential begins with the Ca^{2+} current and subsides as the Ca^{2+} current subsides. Now you step the presynaptic potential from –80 mV to +120 mV and back and obtain the records in B below. Explain this apparently strange result.

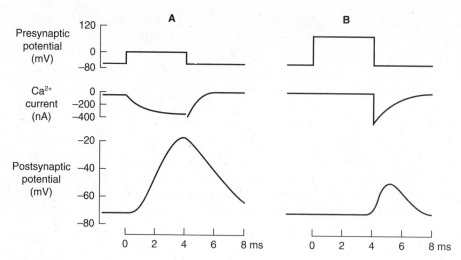

Figure 15–2

You make a new preparation with no TTX or TEA. Assume that you are able to record spontaneous miniature EPSPs (mEPSPs), similar to the spontaneous miniature end-plate potentials recorded at the frog neuromuscular junction in Figure 15–5 in the textbook (p. 275). Assume further that you reduce Ca^{2+} concentration in the bathing medium and record what appears to be quantal variations in the EPSPs evoked by a presynaptic action potential. Like the neuromuscular junction, the presynaptic terminal at the squid giant synapse releases hundreds of vesicles in response to a presynaptic action potential so quantal fluctuations in the EPSP are only apparent with low external Ca^{2+} concentration.

You are able to measure the amplitude of the evoked EPSP and both the amplitude and frequency of the spontaneous mEPSPs accurately.

(g)   What effect will injection of the presynaptic terminal with botulinum toxin have on the evoked EPSP and spontaneous mEPSPs? Why?

(h)   What effect will adding prostigmine and adding curare to the bathing medium have on the evoked EPSP and spontaneous mEPSPs? Why?

(i)   What effect will replacing half of the Na^+ in the bathing medium with an impermeant ion have on the evoked EPSP and spontaneous mEPSPs? Why?

(j)   What effect would injection of IP_3 into the presynaptic terminal have on the spontaneous mEPSPs? Why?

(k) What effect would kandelotoxin have on the spontaneous mEPSPs? Why?

(l) What effect will adding TEA to the bathing medium have on the evoked EPSP and spontaneous mEPSPs, respectively? Why?

4. Review Box 15–1 in the textbook, p. 277. Assume that you have a synapse with $p = 0.1$ and $n = 5$. What effect would doubling the probability of release (the probability of reloading a release site after an action potential and the probability that an action potential discharges a quantum from an active site) from $p = 0.1$ to $p = 0.2$ (the number of loaded release sites $n = 5$) have on the expected number of failures, unit responses, double responses, triple responses, quadruple responses, and quintuple responses in 100 trials and on the (average) quantal content? What effect would decreasing the releasable store of quanta n from 5 to 4 ($p = 0.1$) have on the expected number of failures, unit responses, double responses, triple responses, quadruple responses, and quintuple responses in 100 trials and on the (average) quantal content? These questions are important because neuromodulators can be expected to affect both n and p.

5. The enzyme horseradish peroxidase (HRP), when introduced into nerve cells, can be visualized in the light and electron microscopes by creating an opaque reaction product with a simple histochemical procedure. If HRP is injected into the muscle of a frog nerve-muscle preparation and the preparation is allowed to rest for several minutes before histological fixation and preparation for electron miscroscopy, then HRP reaction product is observed in a small fraction of synaptic vesicles at the neuromuscular junction. If, however, the muscle is activated during the waiting period by high-frequency stimulation of the motor nerve, then a much larger proportion of vesicles at the neuromuscular junctions will contain the HRP reaction product. Explain.

ANSWERS

▧ COMPLETION PROBLEMS

1. miniature end-plate potential

2. size; shape; miniature end-plate potential

3. size; probability

4. 2,000; 6,000; 300; 10^6

5. integral multiples

6. voltage-gated calcium channels

7. mobilization; fusion pore

8. 1.5; 230

9. clathrin coated pits

10. calcium; mobilization

11. calcium influx; synaptic vesicles

▧ TRUE/FALSE QUESTIONS

1. True

2. False. Presynaptic voltage-gated Ca^{2+} channels at the squid giant synapse inactivate *very slowly* upon depolarization.

3. True

4. False. The short time necessary to increase the Ca^{2+} concentration in the presynaptic terminal during an action potential to reach levels that cause synaptic release *does* contribute significantly to the synaptic delay.

5. True

6. True

7. True

8. False. At the vertebrate neuromuscular junction the unit synaptic potential, representing the release of a single quantum of transmitter, *can* be equated with the spontaneous miniature end-plate potential.

9. True

10. False. Miniature end-plate potentials are affected by the cholinergic drugs prostigmine (which produces increases in amplitude) and curare (which produces decreases in amplitude).

11. False. At the vertebrate neuromuscular junction, in the presence of elevated external Mg^{2+} and reduced external Ca^{2+}, increasing the external Ca^{2+} concentration does *not alter* the size of the unit synaptic potential.

12. True

13. True

14. True

15. False. The exocytosis of transmitter from vesicles *transiently increases* the electrical capacitance of secretory cells.

16. False. Transmitter release at *most* but not all chemical synapses is accomplished by exocytosis from vesicles.

17. True

18. True

19. True

20. True

21. True

22. False. Rab 3 proteins are *GTP*-binding proteins that assist in vesicle docking.

23. True

24. False. Increased Cl^- conductance in presynaptic terminals can *decrease* the amplitude of the action potential and thus cause presynaptic *inhibition*.

25. False. The release machinery itself *can be* modulated by presynaptic neural input to regulate transmitter release.

26. True

27. False. Modulation of action potential duration *is a very effective* way to regulate transmitter release.

■ SYNTHETIC QUESTIONS AND QUANTITATIVE PROBLEMS

1. See Figures 15–12B and 17–7B in the textbook

2. (a)

Tethering	*Filling*	*Docking Complex*
Synapsins	Vesicle transporters	Synaptotagmin (P65)
		VAMPS (synaptobrevin)
		NSF
		a-SNAP, g-SNAP, SNAP-25
		Syntaxins
		Neurexins

Fusion pore	*Targeting*	*Freeing*
Synaptophysin	Rab proteins	Ca^{2+}/calmodulin-dependent
Physophillin		protein kinase

Recycling
Clathrin

   (b)   Botulinum toxin — VAMPs (synaptobrevin)

   Tetanus toxin — VAMPs (synaptobrevin)

   a-latrotoxin — Neurexins

3. (a)   Replacing Ca^{2+} ions with Co^{2+} ions in the bathing medium would block the EPSP but not the ACh response. Calcium entry into the presynaptic terminal through voltage-gated Ca^{2+} channels (which are blocked by Co^{2+}) is necessary for transmitter release and thus for the EPSP, but no Ca^{2+} is necessary for the ACh response.

   (b)   Injecting the presynaptic terminal with botulinum toxin will block the EPSP because it interferes with the mechanism of release of transmitter vesicles (enzymatic cleaving of VAMPs).

   (c)   Prostigmine will augment and prolong the EPSP and the ACh response, because it prolongs the lifetime of ACh at the post-synaptic ACh receptors by blocking their destruction by acetyl-cholinesterase. Curare will block (or at least reduce) both the EPSP and the ACh response, because it will block (or at least partially block) the postsynaptic ACh receptors.

   (d)   Replacing half of the Na$^+$ in the bathing medium with an imper-meant ion will reduce the amplitude of both the EPSP and the ACh response. The ACh receptor-channels are permeable to both

Na$^+$ and K$^+$, and the reversal potential of the ACh response and the EPSP is approximately 0 mV under normal conditions. Reducing external Na$^+$ will make the reversal potential more negative and thus reduce both the EPSP and the ACh response.

(e) Kandelotoxin could interfere with presynaptic transmitter release either by blocking Ca^{2+} entry or interfering with the intracellular release machinery. A presynaptic mode of action is indicated because the ACh response is unaltered by kandelotoxin, thus showing that the toxin does not interfere with postsynaptic mechanisms.

(f) When you step the presynaptic potential from –80 mV to +120 mV you activate the presynaptic voltage-gated Ca^{2+} channels strongly, but no Ca^{2+} current flows because at +120 mV you are very near the equilibrium potential for Ca^{2+}. Because no Ca^{2+} current flows during the depolarizing step, there is no synaptic release and thus no postsynaptic potential. When you step back to –80 mV from +120 mV, Ca^{2+} current flows transiently because the Ca^{2+} channels take time to turn off (deactivate) and the inward driving force for Ca^{2+} is restored. During this transient Ca^{2+} current flow there is synaptic release and hence a transient postsynaptic potential.

(g) Injecting the presynaptic terminal with botulinum toxin will block both the evoked EPSP and spontaneous mEPSPs because it interferes with the release mechanism for transmitter vesicles (enzymatic cleaving of VAMPs).

(h) Prostigmine will augment and prolong the evoked EPSP and the spontaneous mEPSPs because it prolongs the lifetime of ACh at the postsynaptic ACh receptors by blocking their destruction by acetylcholinesterase. Curare will block (or at least reduce) both the evoked EPSP and the spontaneous mEPSPs because it will block (or at least partially block) the postsynaptic ACh receptors.

(i) Replacing half of the Na$^+$ in the bathing medium with an impermeant ion will reduce the amplitude of both the evoked EPSP and the spontaneous mEPSPs. The ACh receptor-channels are permeable to both Na$^+$ and K$^+$ and the reversal potential of both the evoked EPSP and the spontaneous mEPSPs is approximately 0 mV under normal conditions. Reducing external Na$^+$ will make the reversal potential more negative, and thus reduce both the evoked EPSP and the spontaneous mEPSPs.

(j) Injecting IP$_3$ into the presynaptic terminal should release Ca^{2+} from internal stores, thus increasing the internal Ca^{2+} concentration and consequently the frequency of spontaneous mEPSPs.

(k) If kandelotoxin acts by blocking Ca^{2+} entry, it probably will have little effect on the spontaneous mEPSPs, which occur even when Ca^{2+} entry is restricted by elevated external Mg^{2+} levels. If kandelotoxin acts by interfering with the intracellular release machinery, it will probably block spontaneous mEPSPs.

(l) Adding just TEA to the bathing medium will augment and prolong the evoked EPSP and have little or no effect on the spontaneous mEPSPs. TEA will broaden the presynaptic action potential because voltage-gated K^+ channels will no longer contribute to the repolarization of the spike (repolarization is achieved by inactivation of the voltage-gated Na^+ channels and current through the leakage channels). The broadened action potential will more effectively and persistently activate the presynaptic voltage-gated Ca^{2+} channels, thus augmenting and prolonging Ca^{2+} entry and consequently synaptic release. TEA should have no effect on the spontaneous release of transmitter quanta or on the response of the muscle membrane to evoked or spontaneous release of transmitter.

4. Under normal conditions ($n = 5$, $p = 0.1$), you expect 59 failures, 33 unit responses, 7 double responses, 0 triple responses, 0 quadruple responses, and 0 quintuple responses in 100 trials, and the (average) quantal content ($m = pn$) will be 0.5.
    With elevated p ($n = 5$, $p = 0.2$), you expect 33 failures, 41 unit responses, 20 double responses, 5 triple responses, 1 quadruple response, and 0 quintuple responses in 100 trials, and the (average) quantal content ($m = pn$) will be 1.0.
    With decreased n ($n = 4$, $p = 0.1$), you expect 66 failures, 29 unit responses, 5 double responses, 0 triple responses, 0 quadruple response, and 0 quintuple responses in 100 trials, and the (average) quantal content ($m = pn$) will be 0.4.

5. Horseradish peroxidase enters synaptic vesicles when the vesicles are recycled by endocytosis. In the resting nerve-muscle preparation the only release of synaptic vesicles is spontaneous release of single vesicles, giving rise to miniature end-plate potentials in the muscle. Since only a relatively small number of vesicles are used and recycled, only a small proportion of all the vesicles in the presynaptic terminals of the motor end-plate will contain HRP reaction product. In contrast, in the stimulated preparation large numbers of vesicles are released and recycled because of the constant activity in the presynaptic motor neurons, so a large proportion of vesicles are recycled and contain the HRP reaction product.

16

Neurotransmitters

Overview

Two types of molecules act as neurotransmitters: small molecules and neuroactive peptides. A limited number (nine) of small molecules are known to act as transmitters and most of these are charged molecules, amines, amino acids and their derivatives. Some of these molecules are synthesized solely for use as transmitters (e.g., dopamine and serotonin), while others are common cellular metabolites (e.g., glycine and glutamate). These molecules are synthesized in short biosynthetic pathways by cytoplasmic enzymes that are often specifically expressed in neurons that utilize these transmitters. They are synthesized near their point of release in the presynaptic terminals and then transported into vesicles for release by specific transport proteins. After releasing their contents by exocytosis, vesicles are rapidly refilled once they are recycled (by endocytosis) from the presynaptic membrane.

Large numbers of peptides act as transmitters; groups of these peptides have closely related amino acid sequences and constitute recognizable neuropeptide families. Neuroactive peptides are synthesized in the same fashion that all secretory proteins are synthesized by cells (on ribosomes on the rough endoplasmic reticulum, while being co-translationally transported into the endoplasmic reticulum lumen). They are synthesized as polyproteins containing a few to several, often repeated, neuropeptide sequences.

As polyproteins move through the endoplasmic reticulum and the

Golgi apparatus they are processed by specific proteases into neuropeptides and packaged into specialized secretory vesicles for rapid axoplasmic transport to presynaptic terminals for release. Once the contents of these vesicles are released they cannot be refilled in the terminals, but must be transported back to the cell body for recycling through the Golgi and refilling. Often both a small-molecule transmitter and a peptide are co-released by the presynaptic terminals of a neuron, but it appears that they are released in separate vesicles and possibly by different molecular mechanisms. (ATP is contained in all vesicles; it is released during exocytosis. It, or its metabolites, can act as transmitters if the appropriate postsynaptic receptors are nearby.)

Three mechanisms exist for the removal of transmitters from the synaptic cleft: diffusion in the extracellular space, destruction by a specific enzyme, and reuptake into neurons or glia by specific transporter proteins. Diffusion aids the removal of all transmitters to a certain extent but is particularly important in some cases (e.g., certain peptides). Degradation as a removal mechanism in the synaptic cleft is limited to cholinergic and peptidergic transmission. The enzyme acetylcholinesterase rapidly breaks down ACh released at the neuromuscular junction and central synapses into choline and acetate. Enzymatic proteolysis appears to be important for the removal of neuropeptides, but the specificity of this process is only just beginning to be explored. Reuptake is the predominant method for removal of small molecule transmitters from the synaptic cleft. Specific transporter proteins in the presynaptic terminals or nearby glial cells take up the released molecules with high affinity and recycle them for reuse. There is even such a transporter to recycle choline at the neuromuscular junction and central cholinergic synapses. The importance of these transporters for normal neuronal function is emphasized by the dramatic effects of drugs that block their function. For example, the psychoactive drug cocaine blocks the reuptake of norepinephrine, and the widely used antidepressant Prozac blocks the reuptake of serotonin.

Objectives

1. Understanding the major small-molecule transmitters, their biosynthetic pathways, and their packaging into vesicles for release.

2. Understanding the importance of neuroactive peptides, their synthesis as secretory polyproteins, and their processing and packaging into vesicles by the endoplasmic reticulum and Golgi apparatus for transport and release.

3. Understanding the functional implications of the different sites of synthesis of small-molecule transmitters (by cytoplasmic enzymes) and neuropeptide transmitters (as secretory polyproteins).

4. Understanding the mechanisms for removal of transmitters from the synaptic cleft.

▣ *TRUE/FALSE QUESTIONS*
(If false, explain why)

1. ATP is not a recognized neurotransmitter. _____

2. Acetylcholine is one of the few uncharged neurotransmitters. _____

3. Glutamate is relatively abundant in the cytoplasm of all neurons. _____

4. The term *purinergic* refers to synapses that use histamine as a transmitter. _____

5. Small-molecule transmitters are often trapped inside vesicles at high concentration because they are kept in a charged state by the transport of proton into the vesicles. _____

6. The enzymes that synthesize small-molecule transmitters are synthesized on free (cytosolic) polyribosomes in the cell body and distributed throughout neurons by slow axoplasmic transport. _____

7. Some neuroactive peptide transmitters are also hormones acting on non-neural tissues. _____

8. Neuroactive peptides are derived from secretory polyproteins and are processed by the major membrane system of the cell, the endoplasmic reticulum and Golgi apparatus. _____

9. Neuroactive peptides are grouped into families based on their physiological effects. _____

10. The specific proteases that process polyproteins into neuroactive peptides in the Golgi apparatus are usually proline proteases. _____

11. The processing of a polyprotein into neuroactive peptide(s) takes place in the cytoplasm. _____

12. More than one copy of the same peptide can be produced from one polyprotein. _____

13. The genes that encode the polyproteins destined to become neuroactive peptides can be alternatively spliced during transcription. Thus, different cells expressing the same peptide gene can produce and release a different compliment of neuroactive peptides. _____

14. Neuroactive peptides and small-molecule transmitters are seldom co-released by the same neuron. _____

15. Monoamine oxidase is an enzyme that is important for the destruction of amine transmitters in the synaptic cleft. _____

16. Acetylcholinesterase breaks down ACh at the mammalian neuromuscular junction, thus rapidly punctuating transmission at this synapse. _____

17. The transporter molecules involved in the high-affinity reuptake of released neurotransmitters belong to a superfamily, all members of which are integral membrane proteins that span the membrane six times. _____

18. The binding constant of transporter molecules involved in the high affinity reuptake of released neurotransmitters is typically 25 µM or less. _____

19. Diffusion is not an important mechanism for the removal of neuroactive peptides from the synaptic cleft. _____

SYNTHETIC QUESTIONS AND QUANTITATIVE PROBLEMS

1. Fill in the missing entries in the table below.

Transmitter	Enzyme
_____	Choline acetyltransferase (specific)
Biogenic amines	
_____	Tyrosine hydroxylase (specific)
Norepinephrine	Tyrosine hydroxylase and _____ (specific)
Epinephrine	_____ and _____ (specific)
_____	Tryptophan hydroxylase (specific)
_____	Histidne decarboxylase (specificity uncertain)
Amino acids	
γ-Aminobutyric acid	_____ (probably specific)
Glycine	_____
Glutamate	_____

2. List the four criteria that must be met before a substance is accepted as a neurotransmitter.

3. At the neuromuscular junctions of the crayfish certain motor neurons use both the small-molecule transmitter glutamate and a peptide called proctolin, while other motor neurons innervating the same muscle fibers use only glutamate. In crayfish and other invertebrates muscle fibers may be innervated by more than one motor neuron. The release of glutamate by the motor neurons causes a rapid EPSP in the muscle fibers that leads to a transient increase in muscle tension, without the necessity of an action potential being produced in the muscle fiber (in fact, the particular muscle fibers in question are incapable of producing action potentials). A rapid series of spikes in the motor neuron that does not use proctolin (motor neuron A) causes a rapid series of EPSPs, each of which gives rise to a twitch-like increase in tension that rapidly declines after cessation of spike activ-

ity in the motor neuron.

Curiously, in crayfish, if the axon of a motor neuron is cut, the distal part of the axon that is disconnected from the cell body remains viable for months. The severed axon is able to produce action potentials when stimulated electrically and maintains its synapses with the muscle.

If motor neurons A and B are severed and the distal axon is stimulated, the response of the muscle shows the normal pattern described above for motor neurons A and B respectively. If, however, the axons are severed and the motor neurons are tested a month later, the response to stimulation of motor neuron B becomes identical to that of motor neuron A. Explain.

4. Transmitters and the enzymes that synthesize them can be detected immunohistochemically with specific antibodies. Assume that you have raised a bank of antibodies, each one directed against one of the enzymes in the biochemical pathway from tyrosine to epinephrine, i.e., you have antibodies to tyrosine hydroxylase, aromatic amino acid decarboxylase (L-DOPA decarboxylase), dopamine β-hydroxylase, pteridine reductase, and phenylethanolamine-N-methyltransferase. For each of these antibodies, predict the transmitter type of all the neurons labeled. (Normally, both neurons that use norepinephrine and those that use epinephrine are both called adrenergic. For the purpose of answering this question, call them noradrenergic and adrenergic, respectively.)

5. How is it that GABA-ergic inhibitory motor neurons and glutamatergic excitatory motor neurons in lobsters contain equal amounts (concentrations) of glutamate?

6. What is meant by co-transmission in reference to synaptic transmission? Give an example.

ANSWERS

■ *TRUE/FALSE QUESTIONS*

1. False. ATP *is* a recognized neurotransmitter.

2. False. Acetylcholine is a *charged* neurotransmitter.

3. True

4. False. The term "purinergic" refers to synapses that use *ATP or its metabolites* as transmitters.

5. True

6. True

7. True

8. True

9. False. Neuroactive peptides are grouped into families based on their *amino acid sequence and gene structure and sequence.*

10. False. The specific proteases that process polyproteins into neuroactive peptides in the Golgi apparatus are usually *serine* proteases.

11. False. The processing of *a* polyprotein into neuroactive peptide(s) takes place inside *membrane-bounded compartments* (endoplasmic reticulum, Golgi apparatus, and transport and secretory vesicles).

12. True

13. True

14. False. Neuroactive peptides and small-molecule transmitters are *often* co-released by the same neuron.

15. False. Monoamine oxidase is an enzyme that degrades amine transmitters within the cell and is *not* important for the destruction of amine transmitters in the synaptic cleft.

16. True

17. False. The transporter molecules involved in the high-affinity reuptake of released neurotransmitters belong to a superfamily, all members of which are integral membrane proteins that span the membrane *twelve* times.

18. True

19. False. Diffusion is thought to be an *important* mechanism for the removal of neuroactive peptides from the synaptic cleft.

■ SYNTHETIC QUESTIONS AND QUANTITATIVE PROBLEMS

1. See Table 16–1 in the textbook, p. 294.

2. (i) The substance is synthesized in the neuron. (ii) The substance is present in the presynaptic terminal and is released in amounts sufficient to exert a defined action on the postsynaptic neuron or effector organ. (iii) When administered exogenously in reasonable concentrations, the substance exactly mimics the action of the endogenously released transmitter (e.g., it activates the same ion channels or second-messenger pathway in the postsynaptic neuron). (iv) A specific mechanism exists for removing the substance from its site of action (synaptic cleft).

3. The rapid increase in twitch-like tension in response to each action potential in either motor neuron A or B is probably due to the observed EPSPs brought about by the release of glutamate with each action potential in the motor neurons. The long-lasting increase in tension produced by activity in motor neuron B is probably due to the

long-lasting muscle depolarization after the EPSPs, which is brought about by the release of proctolin by sustained activity in motor neuron B. Immediately after the axons are severed this normal physiology is observed. If the axons have been severed for a month before testing, then proctolin is probably depleted from the severed axon of motor neuron B; therefore, no proctolin effects are observed after motor neuron B stimulation. The depletion is probably due to spontaneous release of vesicles containing proctolin; these vesicles cannot be replenished because neuropeptides are synthesized and packaged in vesicles in the cell body and then transported down the axon to the neuromuscular junction. Glutamate is available in the cytoplasm and the vesicles containing it can be refilled in the presynaptic terminals.

If this hypothesis is correct and an antibody to proctolin is available for immunohistochemical detection of proctolin, then one would expect that newly severed axons of motor neuron B would stain for proctolin, while severed motor neuron B axons would not stain one month later. In fact, this prediction has been confirmed immunohistochemically.

4. (i)   Tyrosine hydroxylase: dopaminergic, noradrenergic, and adrenergic neurons.
   (ii) Aromatic amino acid decarboxylase: dopaminergic, noradrenergic, and adrenergic neurons. (The antibody should also label serotonergic neurons, since it appears that L-DOPA decarboxylase and 5-hydroxy-tryptophan decarboxylase are identical, hence the generic name aromatic amino acid decarboxylase. Similar enzymes might also be present in other neurons.)
   (iii) Pteridine reductase: all neurons.
   (iv) Dopamine β-hydroxylase: noradrenergic and adrenergic neurons.
   (v)   Phenylethanolamine-N-methyltransferase: adrenergic neurons.

5. Apparently the glutamatergic motor neurons possess proteins (e.g., enzymes and transporters) that allow them to package metabolically generated glutamate into vesicles for release, while GABA-ergic motor neurons lack these proteins.

6. Co-transmission occurs when more than one chemical substance is released by a neuron at its synapses and these molecules have effects on postsynaptic targets. Many mammalian motor neurons release both the small-molecule transmitter ACh and the neuropeptide CGRP. The ACh binds to nicotinic ACh receptors and gate these channels open, thus depolarizing the muscle. CGRP binds to receptors coupled to adenylyl cyclase, raising cAMP and cAMP-dependent protein phosphorylation in the muscle, leading to an increase in the force of muscle contraction.

17

A Clinical Example: Myasthenia Gravis

Overview

The classical form of myasthenia gravis is an autoimmune disease that affects synaptic transmission at the neuromuscular junction. To understand the etiology of the disease it is necessary to understand the basic mechanisms of synaptic transmission at the neuromuscular junction. Circulating antibodies to the nicotinic ACh receptor of the neuromuscular junction, usually directed against a specific area of the α subunit of the receptor, bind to the receptors, thus cross-linking the receptors and increasing their rate of turnover and degradation. Thus, there are fewer functional receptors at the neuromuscular junction in myasthenic patients than normal. Moreover, the postjunctional folds of the muscle membrane are reduced and the synaptic cleft widened, probably because antireceptor antibody activates the complement cascade, which causes focal lysis or breakdown of the postsynaptic membrane.

This reduction in receptors and deterioration of the postsynaptic membrane specialization reduces the amplitude of the end-plate potential evoked by an action potential in the presynaptic motor neuron. Because the end-plate potential must exceed threshold for an action potential if muscle contraction is to result, the safety factor for faithful transmission across the junction becomes reduced. Thus, the repeated activity in motor neurons, which produces movements, is not faithfully transmitted.

Failures to evoke a postsynaptic (muscle) action potential then occur, because random fluctuations in the number of transmitter quanta released can often cause the myasthenic end-plate potential to fall below threshold. The result is grave muscle weakness.

The symptoms of myasthenia gravis are alleviated by treatment with neostigmine, a potent anticholinesterase. Neostigmine prolongs the action of ACh in the synaptic cleft by preventing its breakdown, and augments and prolongs the abnormally small end-plate potential of myasthenic patients, thus increasing the safety factor and the faithfulness of neuromuscular transmission. A useful animal model for the study of myasthenia gravis can be produced by immunizing mice against purified nicotinic ACh receptors. It has now been realized that not all recognized forms of myasthenia fit this autoimmune model; indeed, some of these disease forms may result from defects in the presynaptic terminals at the neuromuscular junction, defects in cholinesterase, or functional defects in the ACh receptors.

Objectives

1. Understanding how knowledge of the basic cellular mechanisms of neuronal functional is invaluable in elucidating the etiology of neurological disease.

2. Understanding how clinical observation can contribute significantly to our understanding of neuronal function.

■ *TRUE/FALSE QUESTIONS*
(If false, explain why)

1. The safety factor of the end-plate potential at the mammalian neuro-muscular junction can be quite large; in some cases as much as four times the amount of ACh necessary to reach action potential thresh-old is released. _____

2. The circulating antibodies found in classical autoimmune myasthenia gravis are usually directed against a cytoplasmic domain of the nico-tinic ACh receptor. _____

3. The circulating antibodies found in classical autoimmune myasthenia gravis usually block the ability of ACh to bind to the nicotinic recep-tor. _____

4. The drug curare can alleviate the symptoms of myasthenia gravis. _____

5. In classical autoimmune myasthenia gravis, presynaptic terminals at the neuromuscular junction do not release normal amounts of ACh. _____

6. The reduction in number of ACh receptors at the neuromuscular junc-tion in classical autoimmune myasthenia gravis is due to increased turnover of receptors. _____

7. Immunization of mice with nicotinic ACh receptors from the electric ray, *Torpedo*, can induce myasthenia gravis. _____

8. Experimentally induced autoimmune myasthenia gravis cannot be treated with cholinesterase inhibitors. _____

9. It is possible to use ^{125}I-labeled tetrodotoxin to label and count the number of ACh receptors at the neuromuscular junction. _____

10. Plasmapheresis alleviates the symptoms of classical autoimmune myasthenia gravis. _____

◼ SYNTHETIC QUESTIONS AND QUANTITATIVE PROBLEMS

1. A new hereditary human disease is discovered in which the primary symptom is muscle weakness, very much like myasthenia gravis. Patients with this disease have normal numbers of ACh receptors at the neuromuscular junction as determined biochemically, and the junctional specializations in the muscle membrane appear normal. Physiological experiments on muscle biopsies indicate that the end-plate potential is reduced in these patients. Quantal analysis of the end-plate potential in the biopsies indicates that the number of quanta released is normal, but the size of the single quantal response and spontaneous miniature end-plate potentials is similarly reduced. Propose two alternative causes for the disease, one presynaptic in origin and the other postsynaptic in origin, and propose experiments that can distinguish between them.

ANSWERS

■ TRUE/FALSE QUESTIONS

1. True

2. False. The circulating antibodies found in classic autoimmune myasthenia gravis are usually directed against an *extracellular* domain of the nicotinic ACh receptor.

3. False. The circulating antibodies found in classic autoimmune myasthenia gravis usually do *not* block the ability of ACh to bind to the nicotinic receptor.

4. False. The drug *neostigmine,* which is a cholinesterase inhibitor, can alleviate the symptoms of myasthenia gravis.

5. False. In classic autoimmune myasthenia gravis, presynaptic terminals at the neuromuscular junction *release normal amounts* of ACh.

6. True

7. True

8. False. Experimentally induced autoimmune myasthenia gravis *can* be treated with cholinesterase inhibitors.

9. False. It is possible to use ^{125}I-labeled α-*bungarotoxin* to label and count the number of ACh receptors present at the neuromuscular junction.

10. True

■ *SYNTHETIC QUESTIONS AND QUANTITATIVE PROBLEMS*

1. A possible presynaptic defect could be that synaptic vesicles are not filled with the normal amount of ACh (e.g., because of a defective vesicle transporter for ACh). A possible postsynaptic defect could be a defective receptor, which is less sensitive to ACh or has a reduced single-channel conductance. One could test for a possible decreased sensitivity of the postsynaptic receptors to ACh in afflicted individuals by comparing the responses (e.g., total postsynaptic current measured in voltage clamp) to focal applications of known concentrations of ACh at the neuromuscular junction in muscle biopsies from normal and afflicted patients. One could test for a possible decreased single-channel conductance of the ACh receptor-channels in afflicted individuals by comparing single-channel patch-clamp recordings of the ACh receptor-channels (with ACh in the patch pipette) from normal and afflicted muscle. If either or both of these tests indicate a defect in the receptor, then it has been demonstrated that the disease has a postsynaptic origin, otherwise it is likely the defect is presynaptic.

18

From Nerve Cells to Cognition

Overview

To understand how the human brain works, cellular studies must be integrated with methods derived from cognitive and behavioral psychology, clinical disciplines, and computer science. The major task of this concerted approach, cognitive neural science, is to analyze internal representations, the patterns of neural activity that are associated with mental processes, such as perception and motor planning.

Representations of personal space consist of cortical maps of the body derived from somatic sensory input. Inputs from different parts of the body are channeled to different areas of the cortex in an orderly arrangement. The size of the brain region in which a particular body part is represented is proportional not to the area of the receptor surface of that part, but rather to its density of innervation. These maps are modified by experience—as a body part is used more, the size of its cortical representation increases.

Studies of somatic sensory maps at the cellular level have shown that there are actually multiple maps; each submodality, or quality of somatic sensation, has a separate representation in the primary cortical area. In later stages of cortical processing, information about these distinct qualities of sensation is combined in secondary cortical areas to form integrated and complex perceptions. In association areas, such as the posterior parietal cortex, these perceptions are combined with those from other sensory systems, such as vision, to form integrated images of personal, peripersonal, and extrapersonal space. A critical role of the posterior parietal area is to shift attention to different parts of space.

Objectives

1. Understanding the different approaches of experimental psychology, behaviorism, and cognitive psychology to the study of behavior.

2. Understanding internal representations and the five main approaches used in cognitive neural science to analyze them.

3. Understanding how representations of personal space are determined by the orderly mapping of somatic sensory inputs in the cerebral cortex.

4. Understanding how cortical maps can be modified and the experimental evidence for this form of learning.

5. Understanding how the properties of the receptive field of neurons are used to analyze internal representations at a cellular level.

6. Understanding how columns of cells in the cortex form the elementary functional unit in the cerebral cortex.

7. Understanding how lesions of the posterior parietal cortex produce deficits in internal representations and the critical role of the posterior parietal cortex in attentiveness.

▉ COMPLETION PROBLEMS

1. We remember events because the structure and function of the _____ between neurons are modified by _____.

2. The sense of the texture of objects is called _____. The sense of position and movement of our limbs is called _____.

3. Recorded electrical signals that represent the summed activity of a specific part of the brain in response to a sensory stimulus are called _____.

4. The region on the surface of the skin that excites a cell is referred to as the cell's _____.

5. Tactile perception of the size and shape of an object is referred to as _____.

6. Patients who ignore one side of their body (and sometimes half of the outside world) are said to have _____ syndrome.

7. Penfield found that electrical stimulation of discrete parts of the post-central gyrus produced tactile sensations on the _____ side of the body.

■ MULTIPLE-CHOICE QUESTIONS

1. If a sensory nerve of an adult monkey is cut,

   A. the region of somatosensory cortex that maps the area of skin innervated by that nerve becomes permanently silent.

   B. the areas of skin innervated by that nerve become mapped in other areas of somatosensory cortex.

   C. neighboring areas of skin innervated by intact nerves develop larger representations in the somatosensory cortex.

2. Maps of the skin in the primary somatosensory cortex

   A. cannot be modified after birth.

   B. cannot be modified after the first year of lie.

   C. are modified continuously throughout life.

3. Which of the following is *not* a contributing factor to neglect syndrome?

   A. Loss of memories associated with one side of the body.

   B. Disturbances of selective attention.

   C. Disturbance of processing of visual stimuli.

   D. Loss of touch sensation on one side of the body.

4. Damage to the medial surface of the parietal lobe most likely will impair perception of sensory stimuli from the

   A.   face.

   B.   arms.

   C.   trunk.

   D.   legs.

5. The primary somatic sensory area of the cortex contains four separate maps of the body. Which of the following best describes the differences in these maps?

   A.   Each is a map of one of the four limbs.

   B.   Each receives information about a distinct feature of somatic sensation.

   C.   Neurons in each map use different mechanisms to process inputs.

   D.   All of the above.

■ TRUE/FALSE QUESTIONS
   (If false, explain why)

1. The cellular mechanisms of information processing are different in different regions of the brain. _____

2. The properties of networks of neurons are not necessarily identical to the properties of the constituent cells. _____

3. Neural maps of the body surface in the somatic sensory cortex represent the spatial relationship between body parts but not the relative sizes of the body parts. _____

4. Patients with neglect syndrome are usually aware of their deficit. _____

5. In the primary somatic sensory cortex, columns of cells represent elementary functional units in which inputs from different types of receptors are mixed together. _____

■ MATCHING PROBLEMS

1. Primary somatic sensory cortex (S-I)

   A. sensory receptors

2. Gracile and cuneate nuclei of medulla

   B. first synaptic relay in somatic sensory system

3. Dorsal root ganglion cells

   C. second synaptic relay in somatic sensory system

4. Posterior parietal area of cerebral cortex

   D. third synaptic relay in somatic sensory system

5. Ventral posterior nucleus of thalamus

   E. association area

■ SYNTHETIC QUESTIONS AND QUANTITATIVE PROBLEMS

1. Outline the key features of three historical traditions: experimental psychology, behaviorism, and cognitive psychology. For each tradition, identify a strength and a weakness.

2. What is meant by an internal representation?

3. Identify two important contributions of computer science to cognitive neural science.

4. Explain the difference between the methods used by Marshall and Penfield for mapping the organization of the somatic sensory cortex. Which method tells us more about conscious perception?

5. With respect to the modifiability of cortical maps, what is meant by the statement that "cells that fire together, wire together"?

6. Describe a study of spatial perception in patients with parietal lesions that demonstrated that spatial memory is referenced to the body.

7. Explain why early studies concluded that there was only one large representation of the body in the primary somatosensory cortex.

8. Why does a small lesion in area 1 of the primary somatic sensory cortex impair tactile discrimination, but a small lesion in area 2 impairs stereognosis?

9. What is "syndactyly" and how do the sensory representations associated with this condition differ from normal?

ANSWERS

■ COMPLETION QUESTIONS

1. connections; experience

2. touch; proprioception

3. evoked potentials

4. receptive field

5. stereognosis

6. neglect

7. opposite

■ MULTIPLE-CHOICE QUESTIONS

1. C.

2. C.

3. D.

4. D.

5. B.

■ *TRUE-FALSE QUESTIONS*

1. False. The cellular mechanisms of information processing are *essentially identical* in different regions of the brain.

2. True

3. True

4. False. Patients with neglect syndrome are usually *not* aware of their deficit.

5. False. The columns of cells represent elementary functional units in which all inputs come from a *single class of receptor.*

■ *MATCHING PROBLEMS*

1. D.

2. B.

3. A.

4. E.

5. C.

■ SYNTHETIC QUESTIONS AND QUANTITATIVE PROBLEMS

1. *Experimental psychology*

   - Primarily concerned with sensation

   - Learning and memory can be studied using simple experimental approaches

   - *Strength*: used empirical methods rather than introspection

   - *Weakness:* focus on sensation rather than behavior

   Behaviorism

   - Focus on observable aspects of stimuli and behavior

   - Considered internal processes that intervene between sensory stimuli and behavioral output irrelevant

   - *Strength:* abandoned speculation about mental processes

   - *Weakness:* ignored constructive neural processes inside brain that underlie perception and action

   Cognitive psychology

   - Focus on internal processes that intervene between stimulus and action and that shape perception and behavior

   - Emphasis on internal representation with implication that mental events *can* be studied

   - *Strength:* led to the possibility of studying internal representations as patterns of activity in different brain structures

   - *Weakness:* internal representations are not readily accessible to objective analysis

2. An internal representation is the set of internal neural events that are responsible for shaping perception and action. This may be stored in memory as a characteristic pattern of activity in a specific set of interconnected cells.

3. (1) Computers have made it possible to model the activity of large populations of neurons and to test specific ideas about how complex neural systems might carry out these functions.

(2) Computer science is in many ways analogous to brain science. The methods used to study how computers can be made to act intelligently provide a set of ideas and terminology that is potentially useful for studying cognitive processes.

4. Marshall recorded the changes in activity in the cortex evoked by sensory stimuli on the screen. Penfield stimulated the cortex and asked patients to report what was perceived and where on the body it was perceived. At first glance it would appear that Penfield's studies tell us more about conscious perception, since they depend on patients' reports of what they consciously perceive. However, the stimulation techniques used by Penfield were artificial and probably do not resemble natural patterns of sensation. Therefore, Penfield's results should probably be interpreted cautiously, at least as they apply to conscious perception.

5. There is some evidence that afferent connections to cortical neurons are formed on the basis of correlated firing patterns. That is, when two or more cells fire at the same time, the connections from them and between them will be strengthened in parallel. With respect to somatosensory maps, Merzenich showed that when two fingers are sewn together the normal sharp discontinuity between the representations of the two fingers in the cortex is lost, presumably because all input to the two representations is strongly correlated.

6. Patients in Milan with lesions of the right parietal lobe (producing visual neglect on the left side of visual space) were asked to imagine that they were facing a well-known cathedral in the city's main square. They were able to identify from memory buildings to the right of the cathedral but not those to the left. Then they were asked to imagine they were standing on the steps of the cathedral, facing in the opposite direction. Again they were able to identify only buildings to the right, but these were the same buildings they had previously been unable to remember, because they were on the left. Therefore, spatial memory is referenced to the body.

7. Early studies of the representations in the somatic sensory cortex relied on gross recording and stimulation techniques with large electrode sizes and large stimulation intensities. More recent studies with refined techniques (microelectrodes and very low stimulation intensities) have revealed that there are four separate representations in the primary somatic sensory cortex, each representing different features of touch and proprioceptive information.

8. Sensory information from the skin (tactile stimuli) is processed in area 1, while area 2 receives combined inputs about tactile stimuli and

proprioceptive stimuli. Stereognosis is the ability to distinguish objects by holding and manipulating them. This requires interpreting a combination of information about the surface of the object (derived from tactile receptors) and the shape of the object (indirectly perceived as the shape of the hand).

9. Syndactyly is a congenital condition in which fingers or toes are fused together. Studies show that the representation of this fused hand in the cortex is smaller than normal without a clear differentiation between fingers.

   After the fingers are surgically separated, their representations become normally differentiated and assume their normal size in the cortex.

19

Cognition and the Cortex

Overview

Some of the most compelling evidence for the nature and localization of cognitive functions has come from studies of the association areas of the cerebral cortex, areas concerned with the integration of sensory modalities and the planning of movement. There are three main association areas. The prefrontal association cortex is important for the planning of action. Anatomical, cellular, and behavioral studies of the prefrontal association area in monkeys reveal that specific parts of this area are concerned with storing information for future actions. The parietal-temporal-occipital cortex links sensory information from different modalities to form global perceptions and direct language functions. The limbic association cortex is an extensive region that is important for memory and emotional behavior.

The association areas on the two sides of the brain are to some degree specialized, so that some functions are localized on the right side and some on the left side. This asymmetry of function is revealed most dramatically in patients in whom the corpus callosum is transected to alleviate the symptoms of epilepsy. Studies of these patients reveal that, in many respects, the two hemispheres act independently of each other. In general, the left side of the brain performs better on analytic-linguistic tasks, while the right side performs better on spatial-perceptual problems. This asymmetry of function is associated with considerable asymmetry in anatomical structure.

Parallel-distributed processing models provide a promising approach to understanding how association areas carry out cognitive functions. These models, while not necessarily replicas of neural circuits, illustrate the types of operations that can be carried out by networks of interconnected units.

Objectives

1. Understanding the location and general functions of the three main association areas of the cerebral cortex.

2. Understanding how experimental tasks such as the spatial delayed-response have been used to reveal the cognitive components of the prefrontal area.

3. Understanding the effects of lesions of the parietal and temporal association areas on cognitive functions.

4. Understanding the main functions of each cerebral hemisphere, how studies of patients with transections of the corpus callosum have revealed specialized functions in the two hemispheres, and how anatomical differences between the two sides of the brain might contribute to hemispheric specialization.

5. Understanding parallel-distributed processing models and how they can be used to investigagate cognitive functions of the brain.

■ *COMPLETION PROBLEMS*

1. Regions of the cerebral cortex that are concerned with integrating two or more sensory modalities or with the planning of movement are called _____ areas.

2. The premotor area of frontal cortex is concerned with _____ action, while the prefrontal area is concerned with _____ action.

3. The dorsolateral surface of the frontal lobe is part of the _____ association area, while the orbitofrontal cortex on the inferior surface is part of the _____ association area.

4. Lesions of the left parietal lobe often produce aphasia and _____, while lesions of the right parietal lobe produce _____ syndrome.

5. The structure that links the two hemispheres is called the _____.

6. The planum temporale, a region in the temporal lobe that includes Wernicke's area, has been found to be larger on the _____ side of the brain in 65% of brains.

■ *MULTIPLE-CHOICE QUESTIONS*

1. In the monkey, lesions of the principal sulcus in the frontal lobe produce impairments in the ability to perform

   A. tasks involving shape discrimination.

   B. tasks involving a delayed spatial response.

   C. all tasks involving a spatial response, with or without delay.

   D. all tasks requiring short-term memory.

2. In what regions of the brain is association cortex found?

   A. Temporal cortex.

   B. Parietal cortex.

   C. Occipital cortex.

   D. All of the above.

3. If you know someone is left handed, the side of the brain dominant for language would probably be

   A. the right.

   B. the left.

   C. both right and left (mixed dominance).

   D. either right or left (approximately equal chance).

4. A patient who is left dominant for language has had a complete surgical transection of the corpus callosum. If a picture of a fork is briefly presented in the *right* half of the visual field, the patient will

   A. not be able to name the object, but will be able to choose it from among several different objects by feeling the objects with the left hand.

   B. be able to name the object, but will not be able to choose it from among several different objects by feeling the objects with the left hand.

   C. be able to name the object and also able to choose it from among several different objects by feeling the objects with the left hand.

   D. not be able to name the object or identify it with either hand.

5. A patient who is left dominant for language has had a complete surgical transection of the corpus callosum. If a picture of a fork is briefly presented in the *left* half of the visual field, the patient will

   A. not be able to name the object, but will be able to choose it from among several different objects by feeling the objects with the left hand.

   B. be able to name the object, but will not be able to choose it from among several different objects by feeling the objects with the left hand.

   C. be able to name the object and also able to choose it from among several different objects by feeling the objects with the left hand.

   D. not be able to name the object or identify it with either hand.

6. Deficits in delayed-response tasks are most likely to be associated with lesions in the

   A. posterior parietal cortex.

   B. prefrontal association cortex.

   C. parietal-temporal-occipital association cortex.

   D. limbic association cortex.

TRUE/FALSE QUESTIONS
(If false, explain why)

1. The concept of localization of function implies that a specific function is mediated exclusively by one region of the brain. _____

2. Columnar organization, which is characteristic of sensory areas of cortex, is also present in association areas. _____

3. Patients with lesions of the left hemisphere are often indifferent to their disability, whereas patients with right-sided lesions are often exceptionally upset about their symptoms. _____

4. The crossed auditory pathways are more important for perception than the uncrossed pathways. _____

5. The right side of the brain is unable to process any linguistic inputs. _____

MATCHING PROBLEMS

1. Agnosia   A. lesion of *right* temporal lobe

2. Deficits in delayed-response task   B. lesion of *left* temporal lobe

3. Deficits in speed of learning   C. lesion of principal sulcus
   of visual tasks

4. Inability to inhibit certain   D. lesion of inferior temporal
   motor responses   region

5. Deficits in verbal memory   E. lesion of parietal association
                                                    cortex

6. Deficits in memory of faces   F. lesion of inferior prefrontal
                                                    convexity

■ SYNTHETIC QUESTIONS AND QUANTITATIVE PROBLEMS

1. Distinguish between the functions of the premotor area and the prefrontal area of frontal cortex. Identify the differences between the inputs to these areas and their outputs to other parts of the brain.

2. List the parts of the brain that are considered part of the limbic association cortex.

3. The most important function of the prefrontal association area is to weigh the consequences of future actions and act accordingly. Discuss how studies in monkeys using spatial delayed-response tasks are related to this function.

4. Discuss possible functions of the corpus callosum, as revealed by studies of "split-brain" animals and humans in whom the corpus callosum has been surgically transected.

5. Describe how sodium amytal can be used to determine which side of the brain is dominant for language in a patient.

6. Identify the key differences between layered networks and recurrent networks. Which type of network do you think might be a better analog of brain circuits responsible for long-term memory? Explain your answer.

7. Define what is meant by back-propagation in a layered network. Briefly describe how it works. Do you think such a mechanism can account for development of connections in real nervous systems? Explain your answer.

ANSWERS

■ COMPLETION PROBLEMS

1. association

2. initiating; planning

3. prefrontal; limbic

4. agnosia; neglect

5. corpus callosum

6. left

■ MULTIPLE-CHOICE QUESTIONS

1. B.

2. D.

3. B.

4. B.

5. A.

6. B.

◼ TRUE-FALSE QUESTIONS

1. False. The concept of localization of function implies that certain areas are more concerned with one kind of function than with others.

2. True

3. False. Patients with lesions of the *right* hemisphere are often indifferent to their disability, whereas patients with *left*-sided lesions are often exceptionally upset about their symptoms.

4. True

5. False. The right side of the brain is able to process simple linguistic inputs.

◼ MATCHING PROBLEMS

1. E.

2. C.

3. D.

4. F.

5. B.

6. A.

■ SYNTHETIC QUESTIONS AND QUANTITATIVE PROBLEMS

1. The premotor cortex is important for the initiation of action; the prefrontal area is important for the planning of action. The premotor cortex receives input from other higher-order areas of cortex that are closely connected with primary sensory areas. It sends its output to the primary motor cortex. The prefrontal association cortex receives inputs from other higher-order areas of cortex that are less closely connected with primary sensory areas. It sends its outputs to premotor cortex and therefore influences movement control in a more indirect fashion.

2. The limbic association cortex includes the orbitofrontal cortex, the cingulate region, and the parahippocampal area.

3. Spatial delayed-response tasks measure the ability of animals to use information stored in spatial memory to make a decision regarding an action. Thus lesions of the prefrontal association area that impair this ability demonstrate the importance of these areas in using prior experience to plan future action.

4. Despite the finding that the two hemispheres can act independently, the corpus callosum is necessary to convey learned information between the two hemispheres. This was revealed by Sperry's finding that split-brain monkeys could be trained with visual input to one side of the brain, but could not make use of that training when the input was presented to the opposite visual field. Another function of the corpus callosum is to allow cooperation between the two sides of the brain, especially in activities requiring coordination of both hands. Patients with surgical transections of the corpus callosum sometimes show interference between the two hands.

5. Sodium amytal is a fast-acting barbiturate. When injected into one of the carotid arteries it transiently blocks neural function in the ipsilateral cerebral hemisphere. After a brief period it will spread to the opposite side of the brain, and therefore only the initial loss of function that occurs can be assumed to represent the function of one hemisphere. For example, sodium amytal is injected into the left carotid artery while a patient is asked to speak continuously. If there is an immediate cessation of speaking, the left hemisphere is dominant for language.

6. In a layered network the strengths of the connection between input and output elements are set by computer algorithms (e.g., back-propagation), which determine the optimal strengths needed to achieve the desired behavior of the network. In a recurrent network the strengths of the connections depend on feedback loops that modify the strengths of input elements on the basis of actual output. Recurrent networks probably represent a better analog of long-term memory. Recurrent networks can "learn" to reach a steady state that reflects a particular combination of inputs and feedback. This steady state is essentially an associative memory.

7. Back-propagation is a technique for modifying strengths between connections in a layered network. Given a problem that the network is designed to solve, the algorithm begins with the output elements and works backward to the input elements, successively calculating the connection strengths that would correctly solve the problem. This process is applied iteratively until an optimal set of connection strengths is reached. Although back-propagation is a useful method for optimizing neural network models, it seems unlikely that it mimics the processes in actual neural development, because it depends on prior knowledge of optimal behavior of the network. Newer techniques, termed genetic algorithms, simulate the evolutionary forces that may have determined connection strengths during phylogenesis.

20

The Sensory Systems

Overview

The study of sensory systems requires two modes of analysis: psychophysics, which focuses on quantitative relationships between stimulus characteristics and perception, and sensory physiology, which examines the neural consequences of sensory stimuli. Psychophysics analysis has identified four major attributes of sensation: modality, intensity, duration, and location. Modality, or quality of the sensation, is a property of sensory nerve fibers, in that different nerve fibers are activated by different types of stimuli.

All sensory systems have a common organizational plan. Each has a serial or hierarchical organization. Primary sensory neurons enter the central nervous system and connect to projection or relay nuclei. Each receptor cell, as well as each neuron along the sensory pathway has a defined receptive field, the area on the receptor sheet in which a stimulus can fire that cell. Each sensory system also has a parallel organization: multiple serial pathways carry different submodalities. At each level of information processing in a sensory system the neurons are anatomically organized into neural maps of the receptor surface of the body; that is, the spatial relations of the receptors in the periphery are maintained throughout afferent pathways.

Each attribute of sensation is encoded in neural signals in specific ways. *Modality* is determined by specific processes of stimulus transduction in receptor cells; different types of receptor cells have specialized membrane

211

properties that cause ion channels to open or close in response to specific types of stimulus energies. This type of energy is then encoded as a labeled line code — the perceived quality of the sensation depends on the specific connections that the receptor makes within the central nervous system. *Intensity* of the stimulus is transmitted by a frequency code (the number of action potentials generated by a stimulus per unit time, as well as by a population code (the number of neurons excited by the stimulus). Information about the *duration* of a stimulus is encoded in the discharge patterns of rapidly and slowly adapting receptors. Discrimination of the *location* of a stimulus is sharpened by lateral inhibition at sensory relay nuclei.

Although all sensory systems have a common organization, each has specific anatomical features that influence the processing of information. The somatosensory system consists of a variety of different types of receptors distributed throughout the body. Taste and smell depend on chemoreceptors; they show little evidence of topographic organization but depend critically on population codes. The auditory system maps pressure waves into distinct frequencies and its anatomical organization allows localization of sound in space.

Objectives

1. Understanding the main assumptions underlying the approaches of sensory psychophysics and sensory physiology.

2. Understanding the distinctions between modality, intensity, duration, and location of a sensation, and how each attribute is measured.

3. Understanding the general characteristics of the major types of sensory receptors.

4. Understanding what is meant by receptive field.

5. Understanding the distinction between serial and parallel organization of sensory pathways.

6. Understanding what is meant by neural maps.

7. Understanding the process of stimulus transduction by sensory receptors.

8. Understanding how the main attributes of sensory stimuli—modality, intensity, duration, and location—are encoded by the nervous system.

9. Understanding the distinguishing characteristics of each of the major sensory systems.

COMPLETION PROBLEMS

1. The lowest stimulus intensity a subject can perceive is called the sensory _____. The minimum difference between two stimuli that a subject can perceive is called the _____ difference.

2. The particular type of stimulus energy to which a receptor is sensitive is called the _____ stimulus.

3. Relay nuclei for virtually all sensory pathways to the cerebral cortex are located in the _____.

4. Sensory information is used for four main functions: _____, control of _____, _____ of internal organs, and maintenance of _____.

5. Sensory receptors that respond transiently at the onset or termination of a stimulus are called _____ receptors. Receptors that fire throughout the stimulus are called _____ receptors.

6. The ability to perceive the position or movement of the limbs is called _____.

MULTIPLE-CHOICE QUESTIONS

1. Stimulus intensity is encoded

   A. in the frequency of discharge of primary afferent fibers (frequency code).

   B. by the number of primary afferent fibers activated (population code).

   C. by the type of primary afferent fiber active (labeled line code).

   D. both A and B.

   E. A, B, and C.

2. Which of the following statements best describes peripheral coding mechanisms in the somatic sensory system?

   A. As the intensity of a stimulus becomes greater, individual receptors discharge action potentials of greater magnitude.

   B. As the intensity of a stimulus becomes greater, individual receptors discharge action potentials at higher frequencies and a greater number of receptors are recruited into action.

   C. An individual receptor may be activated by either thermal, mechanical, or noxious stimuli but the pattern of evoked action potentials differs for each of the various stimuli.

3. Stimulus quality (modality) is encoded in the somatosensory system by

   A. pattern coding.

   B. frequency coding.

   C. labeled line coding.

   D. population coding.

4. Applied to the somatosensory system, the term "receptive field" refers to

   A. the set of primary sensory neurons activated by a particular stimulus.

   B. the region on a receptor cell that is specialized for stimulus transduction.

   C. the area in the parietal lobe responsible for somatic perception.

   D. the area of the body where a stimulus will cause a primary sensory neuron to fire.

5. The only sensory modality in which neural pathways bypass the thalamus and project directly to cerebral cortex is

   A. hearing.

   B. taste.

   C. smell.

   D. pain.

   E. vision.

■ TRUE/FALSE QUESTIONS
(If false, explain why)

1. The perceived duration of a stimulus is independent of stimulus strength. _____

2. In all sensory systems the sensory receptor is a neuron. _____

3. The nervous system can distinguish a touch stimulus from a painful stimulus because the two types of stimuli produce differently shaped action potentials in the sensory neurons. _____

4. The receptor potential is a graded response, that is, its amplitude is proportional to the strength of the stimulus. _____

5. Perception of the location of a stimulus in the somatosensory system depends critically on somatotopic organization. _____

■ MATCHING PROBLEMS

1. Stimulus intensity

2. Stimulus duration

3. Sensory modality

4. Stimulus location

5. Selective perception

6. Discrimination between stimuli

A. lateral inhibition

B. somatotopy

C. feed-forward inhibition

D. Weber's law

E. law of specific nerve energies

F. rapidly adapting receptors

▪ SYNTHETIC QUESTIONS AND QUANTITATIVE PROBLEMS

1. When a tree falls in the forest, does it make a sound if no one hears it? Explain your answer.

2. A person may be easily able to distinguish between a 1 kg and a 2 kg weight and yet not be able to distinguish between 50 and 51 kg. Describe the psychophysical principle that quantifies this phenomenon. Speculate as to why this property of sensory systems might be useful.

3. Define what is meant by the terms "sensory modality" and "submodality." Make an outline of the five major sensory modalities and list the important submodalities. For each submodality identify the type of sensory receptor (e.g., mechanoreceptor).

4. List the four major attributes or properties of sensory information. Identify and briefly explain the principal way each property is encoded by the nervous system.

5. Explain why a population code may be needed to supplement a frequency code in encoding intensity as the strength of a stimulus increases.

6. Distinguish between lateral (or feedback) inhibition and feed-forward inhibition. Identify an important function of each type of inhibition.

7. Distinguish between Locke's empiricist view and Kant's idealism as they relate to the study of sensation. Identify the two scientific disciplines that arose from these philosophical ideas and discuss their influence on contemporary neural science.

8. A person who receives a sharp blow to the eye area may "see stars." Explain why such a phenomenon occurs.

9. Define what is meant by two-point threshold. Explain how the ability to discriminate two stimuli on the skin might be enhanced by lateral inhibition.

ANSWERS

◼ COMPLETION QUESTIONS

1. threshold; just noticeable

2. adequate

3. thalamus

4. perception; movement; regulation; arousal

5. rapidly adapting; slowly adapting

6. proprioception

◼ MULTIPLE-CHOICE QUESTIONS

1. D.

2. B.

3. C.

4. D.

5. C.

■ TRUE/FALSE QUESTIONS

1. False. The perceived duration of a stimulus *depends on* stimulus strength.

2. False. In some sensory systems the receptor cell is a *specialized epithelial cell.*

3. False. The nervous system can distinguish the two types of stimuli because they activate *different types of receptors.*

4. True

5. True

■ MATCHING PROBLEMS

1. D.

2. F.

3. E.

4. B.

5. C.

6. A.

■ SYNTHETIC QUESTIONS AND QUANTITATIVE PROBLEMS

1. Although the tree falling creates pressure waves in the air, it does not create a sound. Sound occurs only when the pressure waves are perceived by a living being.

2. The "just noticeable difference" between the two stimuli increases in proportion to the magnitude of the stimuli (Weber's law). This property of sensory systems maximizes the range over which stimuli can be evaluated (from weak to strong) while at the same time allowing very fine discrimination of weak stimuli. If the just noticeable difference was constant and also small, the firing rates of sensory receptors would saturate with strong stimuli.

3. Sensory modality refers to the distinctive quality of a sensation (e.g., sound or taste). Submodality refers to the different qualities of sensation that can be distinguished within each of the major senses (e.g., sweet or sour for taste).

Vision 　　Color 　　Movement	Photoreceptors
Hearing	Mechanoreceptors
Touch 　　Touch 　　Proprioception 　　Temperature 　　Pain	 Mechanoreceptors Mechanoreceptors Thermoreceptors Nociceptors
Taste 　　Sweet 　　Sour 　　Salty 　　Bitter	Chemoreceptors
Smell 　　Many different odors	Chemoreceptors

4. The four major attributes of sensory information are modality, intensity, duration, and location. *Modality* is encoded by a labeled line code. The information from receptors that respond selectively to a given type of physical energy projects to a distinct part of the cerebral cortex. *Intensity* is encoded by a combination of a frequency code and a population code. Higher intensities of stimulation produce higher rates of firing in receptors and activate greater numbers of receptors. *Duration* is encoded by rapidly and slowly adapting receptors. Rapidly adapting receptors increase their firing rate transiently at the onset and offset of a stimulus. Slowly adapting receptors maintain a high firing rate throughout the time a stimulus is presented. *Location* is encoded as the receptive field of a neuron, the area on the receptive sheet in which stimuli cause a change in the neuron's firing rate.

5. A population code, in which more neurons are activated as the strength of a stimulus increases, allows the nervous system to sense very strong stimuli even though the firing rate of individual receptors may be saturated (i.e., reach their maximal rates) with intermediate stimulus strengths.

6. In lateral inhibition, neighboring neurons within a relay nucleus may inhibit a specific neuron. This type of inhibition allows neurons that are receiving a stronger signal to inhibit those that are responding weakly to the stimulus, thus increasing the contrast of a sensation. In feed-forward inhibition, specific relay nuclei of the brain can inhibit certain neurons in other nuclei. This mechanism allows the brain to selectively attend to stimuli that are most important at the moment and to screen out irrelevant stimuli.

7. According to Locke's empiricist view, the human mind is at birth a blank slate that is primarily "filled" by experience. This view was the forerunner of behaviorist psychology, which led to a focus in early neural science on studying observable behavior. Kant's idealism stressed that the human mind has inherent rules and constraints that form a "preknowledge." This view was the forerunner of cognitive psychology, which had led to the current focus in neural science on discovering the neural correlates of internal representations.

8. This phenomenon occurs because the perceived quality or modality of a sensation depends on a labeled line code. When a person receives a sharp blow to the eye area, the high intensity of the mechanical stimulation causes some photoreceptors to respond. However, because the firing of these receptors ultimately projects to the visual areas of the brain, the person perceives the stimuli as changes in light intensity instead of changes in mechanical intensity.

9. A two-point threshold is the smallest distance between two *detectable* stimuli at different points on the skin, such that the two stimuli are perceived as discrete stimuli instead of as one stimulus. Lateral inhibition enhances the contrast between an area of skin that is strongly stimulated and surrounding areas that are only weakly stimulated. When two areas of skin that are close together are simultaneously stimulated, the area between them is weakly stimulated by both stimuli. Without lateral inhibition the two weak stimuli might summate, leading to the perception that the area is actually being strongly stimulated. With lateral inhibition, neurons that respond strongly to the direct stimulation inhibit neurons that respond weakly, allowing the perception that the two stimuli are different.

21

Construction of the Visual Image

Overview

We see things around us effortlessly. For this reason it is often difficult for us to appreciate the enormous complexity involved in processing visual information. A large amount of information is lost when the three-dimensional world is projected two-dimensionally onto two separate retinas. There is simply not enough information in the retinal images to allow a unique reconstruction of the three-dimensional world by the brain. The problem is further complicated by the fact that the retinal images are strongly dependent on some unknown factors such as the precise locations and spectral compositions of the light sources and the orientations and reflectances of the objects in the world. The brain, therefore, has to "guess" at the missing information by making sensible assumptions about the world so that good solutions can be produced rapidly enough under most circumstances. In this sense visual perception is necessarily a creative process. These assumptions about the world are presumably embedded in the neural networks along the visual pathway and they manifest themselves at the behavioral level as *laws of perception* as described by Gestalt psychologists.

Three parallel and interacting pathways have been identified in the primate visual system. They appear to be involved in the processing of motion, form, and color, respectively. The relative separation of different types of visual information in the brain is supported by clinical studies on patients with specific visual deficits. To account for our unified perceptual experiences despite the parcellation of visual information in the brain, it has been suggested that visual attention may help bind together the different visual attributes of the same object processed in separate pathways.

Objectives

1. Understanding the psychological evidence suggesting that visual perception is a creative process.

2. Understanding the overall structure of the major visual processing pathways.

3. Understanding the difference between the pre-attentive and attentive processes as revealed by pop-out experiments.

■ COMPLETION PROBLEMS

1. Visual processing starts at the retina. The axons of the retinal _____ cells project to _____ in the thalamus.

2. The primary visual cortex is also known as _____, _____, and _____. It receives input from _____ and projects to extrastriate areas.

3. There are three relatively separate visual pathways. The parvocellular–blob pathway is mainly concerned with _____ perception. The parvocellular–interblob pathway is mainly concerned with the perception of _____ and _____. The magnocellular–thick stripes pathway is mainly concerned with the perception of _____ and _____.

◼ *MULTIPLE CHOICE QUESTIONS*

1. An equiluminant stimulus used in visual psychophysics

   A. is a uniform monochromatic display.

   B. varies in color but not in brightness distribution.

   C. contains several colored patches.

   D. is ideal for generating motion perception.

2. The pre-attentive process

   A. solves the binding problem.

   B. is just as fast as the attentive process.

   C. can detect the difference in elementary features but not the difference in combinations of the features.

   D. scans individual features in a stimulus sequentially.

3. Cells in the blob regions of V1

   A. are selective to color but not orientation and direction of motion.

   B. are selective to color and orientation but not direction of motion.

   C. project to thick stripes in V2.

   D. receive input from layer 4Cα.

   E. are not as active as cells in the interblob regions.

4. The law of proximity discovered by the Gestalt psychologists states that

   A. when objects are close to each other they appear similar.

   B. the perceived distance between objects is always smaller than the actual distance.

   C. simple features that are close to each other tend to be grouped together perceptually.

   D. nearby cells in the cortex have similar response properties.

■ SYNTHETIC QUESTIONS AND QUANTITATIVE PROBLEMS

1. Consider the situation in the figure below, where each retina contains an image of two dots. To demonstrate that the three-dimensional structure of the world cannot be uniquely determined by the two-dimensional retinal projections, show that at least two different arrangements of dots in space could give rise to the same retinal images.

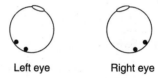

Left eye   Right eye

Figure 21–1

2. In vision research the size of the retinal image generated by an external object is often expressed in terms of the visual angle the object subtends to the eye. The angle is usually expressed in units of degrees or minutes. To gain a sense of these units, determine the retinal image size of your thumb when your arm is fully extended out in front of you.

3. If the parvocellular and magnocellular pathways remained cleanly separated in the extrastriate cortices, what effects on the activities of V4 and MT cells would you expect to observe if you could selectively inactivate either the parvocellular or the magnocellular LGN layers of a monkey?

ANSWERS

■ *COMPLETION PROBLEMS*

1. ganglion; the LGN.

2. V1; area 17; the striate cortex; LGN.

3. color; shape (or form), depth; motion, depth.

■ *MULTIPLE CHOICE QUESTIONS*

1. B.

2. C.

3. A.

4. C.

SYNTHETIC QUESTIONS AND QUANTITATIVE PROBLEMS

1. The retinal images can be generated by dots a and d, or b and c, or b and d and c, etc.

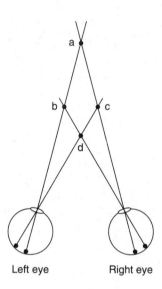

2. The angle is fairly small, and is approximately equal to the size of the thumb divided by the length of the arm. The result so obtained is in radians. To convert it to degrees, multiple the result by $180/\pi$.

3. If the two pathways were entirely separated, one would expect that MT activity should be strongly attenuated by a magnocellular block but not a parvocellular block at LGN, while V4 activity should be attenuated by a parvocellular block but not a magnocellular block. These experiments have been performed by Maunsell and co-workers (J. H. R. Maunsell et al., *J. Neurosci.*, 10, 3323-3334, 1990; A. P. Vincent et al., *Nature*, 358, 756-758, 1992). It was found that MT activity was indeed mainly influenced by the magnocellular block. However, V4 activity was found to depend on both parvocellular and magnocellular inputs.

22

Visual Processing by the Retina

Overview

The light rays from the external world are focused by the cornea and the lens to form images on the retina. The retina contains five major classes of cells: photoreceptors, horizontal cells, bipolar cells, amacrine cells, and ganglion cells. These cells and their processes are well organized into five distinctive layers: outer nuclear, outer plexiform, inner nuclear, inner plexiform, and ganglion cell layers. The light is transduced into electrical signals by the photoreceptors through a cascade of biochemical reactions, involving G-protein and cyclic GMP. The transduction starts with the absorption of light by visual pigments in the photoreceptors and ends with the hyperpolarization of the receptor membrane potential. The simple hyperpolarization is then transformed into the center-surround receptive field organization of the bipolar and ganglion cells by the retinal circuitry. Photoreceptors, horizontal cells, and bipolar cells make synaptic contacts with each other in the outer plexiform layer. Bipolar cells, amacrine cells, and ganglion cells make contacts in the inner plexiform layer.

The two major types of photoreceptors, rod and cones, are responsible for night and day vision, respectively. The cones can be further divided into three types based on their spectral sensitivity. The relative responses of the three types of cones form the basis of color vision. The bipolar and ganglion cells can be classified into on-center and off-center based on their responses to spots of light in the centers of their receptive fields. The response properties of these cells are generated by the specific connectivity among cells in the retina. Most ganglion cells can also be classified into M and P cells according to their sizes. These two types appear to carry different kinds of visual information and they project to different targets in the lateral geniculate body.

Objectives

1. Understanding the anatomical structure of the retina.

2. Understanding the mechanism of phototransduction.

3. Understanding the physiological properties of retinal ganglion cells and their significance in visual information processing.

■ COMPLETION PROBLEMS

1. Of the two types of photoreceptors, _____ are more sensitive to light and therefore are responsible for night vision. _____ mediate color vision because there are _____ types of them, each preferring light of a different frequency range.

2. The central region of the retina, about 5° in diameter, is called the _____. Here visual resolution is _____ due to the high cone density and the lack of blood vessels. Because of constant _____ we are usually unaware of its small size.

3. The region of the retina where the axons of _____ cells exit is called the _____. It forms a "blind spot" because of the lack of the _____ in this region.

4. The visual pigment in rod cells, _____, has two parts. The protein portion is called _____ and the light-absorbing por-

tion is called _____. The absorption of light causes _____ to change from 11-*cis* to _____ configuration, which in turn causes a conformation change in _____.

5. A single activated rhodopsin can trigger the activation of hundreds of _____ molecules. This molecule is a regulatory G-protein, which becomes active through the exchange of _____ for _____. Each G-protein in turn is capable of hydrolyzing more than 10^3 molecules of _____ per second through the activation of the enzyme _____.

6. In the dark, the concentration of cGMP is relatively _____. The concentration of cGMP is _____ by light, causing a _____ of inward Na^+ current through the cGMP-gated channels. This results in _____ of the membrane potential of the photoreceptors.

7. There are about _____ times more rods than cones on the retina. The spatial resolution of the cone system is _____ than that of rod cells because cones cells are highly concentrated in the fovea, where _____ are absent. The temporal resolution of the cone system is also _____ than that of rod cells.

8. Both excitatory and inhibitory synapses are found in the retina. The connection from a cone to an on-center bipolar cell is _____ while that to an off-center bipolar cell is _____. The synapses between the on-center bipolar and on-center ganglion cells are _____.

9. The _____ cells are responsible for the antagonistic surround of bipolar cells.

10. Among the five major classes of retinal neurons, only _____ cells fire action potentials.

11. Most retinal ganglion cells can be classified into two types, _____ and _____, based on their sizes. The _____ cells appear to be concerned with motion analysis while the _____ cells are involved in the perception of color and form.

■ SYNTHETIC QUESTIONS AND QUANTITATIVE PROBLEMS

1. Do a simple experiment on yourself to determine on which side of the fovea the optic disc is located.

2. The light rays entering an eye are bent by both the cornea and the lens to form images on the retina. Contrary to common belief, the cornea actually bends light much more strongly than the lens. (The lens is important for making small adjustments when focusing on objects at different distances, a process called *accommodation*.) Explain why this is the case using the fact that the refraction index of the lens is only slightly larger than that of the surrounding media, while the refraction index of the cornea is much larger than that of the air.

3. Under very dim light one can often see objects better by looking somewhat away from them. Which property of the retina could account for this observation?

4. Part of this page is covered by black ink (to form the text), which reduces the amount of reflected light. The text on the page reflects more light under the sun than the nonprinted part does under a desk lamp, yet the text appears black and the rest of the page white under both lighting conditions. Which property of what types of retinal cells could be used to explain this phenomenon?

5. There are more than 100 million photoreceptors on the retina. The number of retinal ganglion cells, on the other hand, is only around one million. This suggests that there is an over 100-fold compression as signals are passed from photoreceptors to the ganglion cells. Discuss how the compression might be achieved based on the physiological properties of the photoreceptors and the ganglion cells.

6. It has been demonstrated that our visual system can resolve displacement much smaller than the spacing between adjacent photoreceptors in the retina. This phenomenon has been termed hyperacuity. Consider the response properties of the two hypothetical types of photoreceptors in Figure 22–1. In the first case (a) each photoreceptor has an identical response to a given amount of light falling anywhere within its cross section. In the second case (b) the receptor responds in a graded manner to light over an area larger than the size of the receptor. Which system could give rise to hyperacuity and why?

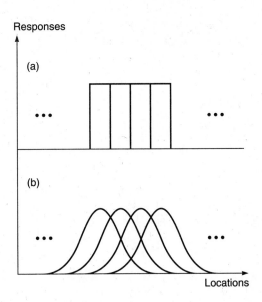

Figure 22–1. Two hypothetical response properties of photoreceptors: (a) no response overlap between adjacent receptors, (b) graded and overlapping responses. Only four photoreceptors for each case are shown.

ANSWERS

◼ COMPLETION PROBLEMS

1. rods; cones; 3

2. fovea; highest; eye movement

3. ganglion; optic disc; photoreceptors

4. rhodopsin; opsin; retinal; retinal; all-trans; opsin

5. transduction; GDP; GTP; cGMP; cGMP photodiesterase

6. high; reduced; reduction; hyperpolarization

7. 20; better; cones; rods; higher

8. inhibitory; excitatory; excitatory

9. horizontal

10. ganglion

11. M; P; M; P

SYNTHETIC QUESTIONS AND QUANTITATIVE PROBLEMS

1. The optic disc is on the nasal side of the fovea. Close your left eye. Extend both of your arms straight in front of you with your two thumbs next to each other and pointing up. Fixate your right eye at the tip of the left thumb while slowly moving the right thumb to the right. You will notice that the tip of the right thumb disappears at some point.

2. Apply Snell's law from optics:

$$n_1 \sin \alpha_1 = n_2 \sin \alpha_2$$

where α_1 and α_2 are the incidence angle and refraction angle, respectively, and n_1 and n_2 are the refraction indices of the two media involved.

3. The rod density is zero at the fovea. It reaches the highest value at about 18° of eccentricity.

4. The center-surround receptive field organization of bipolar and ganglion cells could account for this phenomenon. These cells code contrast rather than light intensity.

5   The photoreceptors code the light intensities at the sampled points in the external world. Because the world is usually composed of many coherent surfaces, light intensities of nearby points in the world are often very similar. Therefore the information carried by photoreceptors is highly redundant. This redundancy is presumably reduced by the ganglion cells, which codes only intensity changes (contrasts) in the visual field.

6. The receptors with graded responses over a larger area (b) could allow the system to have hyperacuity. This is because nearby receptors would be activated to different degrees by a spot of light depending on the location of the spot. The constant and non-overlapping responses shown in (a) could not give rise to hyperacuity because the information on light spot location within the cross section of a receptor is completely lost.

23

Perception of Form and Motion

Overview

The distribution of contrast in retinal images is coded in the firing patterns of retinal ganglion cells. These cells send their outputs to the lateral geniculate nucleus (LGN), which in turn relays the signals to the primary visual cortex (also known as striate cortex, area 17, or V1).

The physiological properties of LGN cells are similar to those of the retinal ganglion cells; they have a center-surround receptive field organization. The representation of visual information is significantly transformed at V1, where most cells respond preferentially to short line segments of a specific orientation. V1 is organized into (1) a retinotopic map, (2) orientation-specific columns, (3) ocular dominance columns, and (4) in the superficial layers color-sensitive blobs. Along the direction perpendicular to the cortical surface, V1 is organized into functionally distinct layers of cells devoted to the processing of motion, color, or form. Thus each layer of cells receives different inputs from LGN and projects to different targets in extrastriate cortex. These two relatively separate processing streams are known as the *where* and *what* pathways, respectively.

Many cells in layers 4B and 6 of V1 are directionally selective. Layer 4B projects to the middle temporal (MT) area, where almost all cells have directional selectivity. MT is organized into a retinotopic map and motion direction-specific columns. Physiological recordings and lesion and microstimulation studies all indicate that MT is important for analysis of motion in the visual field.

Objectives

1. Understanding the structural organizations of LGN and V1, and the physiological properties of the cells in these areas.

2. Understanding the main differences in the organization of the receptive fields of LGN cells and V1 cells.

3. Understanding how the receptive fields of V1 cells transform visual information.

4. Understanding the anatomical and physiological distinctions between the *what* and *where* pathways.

▦ COMPLETION PROBLEMS

1. In primates the LGN contains _____ layers of cell bodies, numbered from the ventral to the dorsal end. Layers number _____ receive input from the ipsilateral eye while layers number _____ receive input from the contralateral eye.

2. The two most ventral layers of LGN are called _____ layers because they contain relatively large cells. These layers receive their inputs from the _____ cells in the retina. The remaining layers are known as the _____ layers, which receive their input from the _____ cells in the retina.

3. The magnocellular cells of LGN send their output to layer _____ of the striate cortex, which then projects to layer _____ of the same area. The parvocellular cells of LGN send their outputs to layers _____ of the striate cortex.

4. Those regions in layers _____ of V1 that stain more heavily for cytochrome oxidase are called blobs. Cells in blobs are selective for _____.

5. Unlike most other cells in V1, cells in layer 4C and in the blob regions of the superficial layers are not _____ selective. These cells receive direct ascending inputs from _____.

6. Cells that prefer line segments of a limited length are called _____ cells.

7. Long-range horizontal connections of V1 cells communicate with other cells of the _____ orientation and color selectivity.

8. At each stage of visual processing, from the retina to LGN to V1 and to extrastriate areas, the receptive field of cells becomes _____, and the response properties become more _____.

9. Areas MT and MST are distinctive in that almost all cells in these areas are highly selective for _____.

10. Cells in the _____ area are best driven by stimuli of complex forms such as faces.

SYNTHETIC QUESTIONS AND QUANTITATIVE PROBLEMS

1. Discuss the main differences and similarities between simple and complex cells in the primary visual cortex.

2. Consider the situation illustrated below, where both eyes are fixating at point *f* in space. To which hemisphere of V1 do the retinal images of points *a*, *b*, and *c* project? If the optic chiasm is damaged, which retinal images of which points will fail to reach LGN?

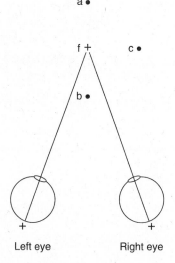

Figure 23–1

3. Changes in light intensity often occur across the boundaries of objects in the world. They can also be caused by the shadows on the objects. We normally have no trouble in distinguishing these two types of intensity changes. Can the orientation-selective cells in V1, with receptive fields similar to those depicted in Figure 23–9B in the textbook (p. 434), distinguish the two types of intensity changes?

4. Give one example for each of the following situations: (1) the retinal image moves and we sense the motion, (2) the retinal image moves but we do not sense any motion, (3) the retinal image is stationary but we sense motion, and (4) the retinal image is stationary and the eye is moving but we do not sense any motion.

5. Consider a wheel with *n* evenly spaced spokes, rotating at an angular speed of ω degrees per second. Suppose snap shots are taken from the wheel every Δ*t* seconds and the resulting frames are shown one after another to create an apparent motion display. (1) Find the relationship between the two ω that will generate the same apparent speed of rotation in the apparent motion display. (2) Determine the conditions under which the wheel appears to rotate in the opposite direction of its true motion. (3) A bike has tires 28 inches in diameter, and each tire has 20 evenly distributed spokes around it. Assuming that the bike is being filmed at the rate of 60 frames per second, at what speed (miles per hour) intervals must the bike move to ensure that the tires appear to rotate in the proper direction in the movie?

6. Suppose you are recording a cell in the inferior temporal cortex and find that it responds most vigorously to an image of your face. What would you do to find out whether the cell really "likes" your face as a whole, or if it is merely driven by some simpler features present in the image?

ANSWERS

■ COMPLETION PROBLEMS

1. 6; 2, 3 and 5; 1, 4 and 6.

2. magnocellular; M; parvocellular; P.

3. 4Cα; 4B; 4Cβ, 2 and 3.

4. 2 and 3; color.

5. orientation; LGN.

6. end-stopped.

7. same.

8. larger; complex.

9. direction.

10. inferotemporal

SYNTHETIC QUESTIONS AND QUANTITATIVE PROBLEMS

1. Simple cells have well-defined excitatory and inhibitory regions in their receptive fields, whereas complex cells do not. Simple cells are located closer to the input layer 4C and have relatively smaller receptive field sizes than do complex cells. Both types of cells are usually selective for orientation and subpopulations of both types are directionally selective or end-stopped.

2. The left and right retinal images of point *a* project to the V1 in the right and left hemispheres, respectively. The left and right retinal images of point *b* project to the V1 in the left and right hemispheres, respectively. Both the left and right retinal images of point *c* project to the V1 in the left hemisphere. If the optic chiasm is damaged, both the left and right retinal images of point *a* and the right retinal image of point *c* will not reach the level of LGN.

3. No.

4. Here are some examples among many possibilities. (1) Fixate at your left thumb while moving your right hand back and forth. (2) Move your eyes or head or body around in a static environment. (3) Move a lit cigarette back and forth in an otherwise completely dark room and follow the cigarette via smooth pursuit eye movement. (4) Fixate at a stationary and lit cigarette in an otherwise completely dark room while turning your head back and forth.*

5. (1)   All ω that differ by integer multiples of $360/n\Delta t$ degrees per second (or equivalently $2\pi/n\Delta t$ radians per second) will generate the same apparent speed of rotation in the apparent motion display.

---

*The head movement generates an equal and opposite eye movement through a process known as the vestibular-ocular reflex. Therefore the retinal image of the cigarette does not move.

(2) For any integer $k = 0, 1, 2, \ldots$, the wheel will appear to rotate in the proper direction when

$$k\frac{360}{n\Delta t} < \omega < \left(k + \frac{1}{2}\right)\frac{360}{n\Delta t}$$

and the wheel will appear to rotate in the opposite direction when

$$\left(k + \frac{1}{2}\right)\frac{360}{n\Delta t} < \omega < (k + 1)\left(\frac{360}{n\Delta t}\right).$$

(3) The speed intervals over which the tires appear to rotate in the proper direction are:

$$k\,4.8 \text{ m/h} < \text{speed} < \left(k + \frac{1}{2}\right) 4.8 \text{ m/h}$$

where $k = 0, 1, 2, \ldots$. Note that the speed of the bike is equal to the angular speed (radians per second) of the tires times the radius of the tires.

6. You could cut the image of your face into several small pieces, rearrange them so that it does not look like a face any more, and then record from the cell with the scrambled image. You could also show images of small regions of your face, one at a time, and examine whether any region by itself drives the cell. If you do succeed in driving the cell with a certain region, you can then record the cell with progressively simplified drawings for that image region. Fujita and his colleagues used this second approach successfully and found that the inferior temporal cortex is organized into columns, each containing cells responsive to similar visual features more complex than line segments but much simpler than faces (Fujita et al., *Nature* 360, 343-346, 1992).

24

Color

Overview

Like most of our normal perceptual experiences, color vision depends on both the external physical stimulation and internal neural processing. The wavelengths of light rays entering the eyes form the physical basis of color vision. Most properties of our color experience, however, can only be understood by studying the neural mechanisms of color processing.

Color vision is only possible by comparing the responses of at least two types of cones with different spectral sensitivities. A system with a single type of cone with a fixed spectral sensitivity would not be able to discriminate different light wavelengths because a given response can be generated by different combinations of light intensity and wavelength. Human color vision uses three different types of cones, R, G, and B. Lights of different wavelengths generate different response patterns in the three types of cones, which are then interpreted by the brain as having different colors. Different wavelength combinations that generate the same response pattern in the three types of cones will appear to have the same color. That is why any color can be matched by combining appropriate proportions of the three primary colors.

The R, G, and B color channels of the cone system are organized into three color-opponent channels at the levels of retinal ganglion cells and LGN. The opponency is further elaborated in the primary visual cortex, where double-opponent cells are found. These physiological properties can explain the perceptual phenomena of color opponency and simultaneous color contrast.

The spectral composition of the light reflected from a surface depends on both the spectral composition of the light source and the surface reflectance of different wavelengths. The phenomenon of color constancy indicates that the perceived color at a given location is not simply determined by the spectral composition of the reflected light from the location. Instead, the brain appears to combine information from nearby locations to discount variations in the light sources and to approximately compute the surface reflectances, an intrinsic surface property. There is physiological evidence indicating that V4 activity may be the neural basis of color constancy.

Objectives

1. Understanding the essential requirements for achieving color vision.

2. Understanding the key perceptual features of color vision.

3. Understanding the neural substrates for color vision.

■ *COMPLETION PROBLEMS*

1. The human eye is sensitive to light with wavelengths from _____ nm to _____ nm.

2. The full spectrum of perceived colors can be matched by combining appropriate proportions of the _____. This results from the fact that there are _____ types of cones, each with a different pigment.

3. Like the rod pigment rhodopsin, the cone pigments are composed of a protein called _____ and the light-sensitive compounds called _____. There are three types of cone pigments, each containing a different _____.

4. There are three color opponent channels: _____,
   _____, and _____.

5. The red-green double-opponent cells can be best driven by
   _____ color in the center and _____ color in the
   surround of the receptive fields.

6. The R and G pigments genes are located on the _____ chromosome and are next to each other. The B pigment gene is on the
   _____ chromosome and the rhodopsin gene is on the
   _____ chromosome.

■ MULTIPLE CHOICE QUESTIONS

1. If someone suddenly lost all his short and middle wavelength cones,

   A.   the world would appear red to him.

   B.   he would not be able to see anything.

   C.   he could only see under very dim light.

   D.   the world would appear gray to him.

2. A sheet of red paper appears red to us because

   A.   it absorbs red light.

   B.   it emits red light.

   C.   it absorbs less red light and reflects more red light than all other
        lights.

   D.   it does not reflect red light away.

3. We do not see color under dim light because

   A.   rods are equally sensitive to lights of all wavelength.

   B.   the rod system has poor spatial and temporal resolution.

   C.   the reflected light from objects contains equal proportions of all
        wavelengths.

   D.   there is only one type of rod.

4. The fact that a green object stands out more against a red than a blue background

    A. is because the wavelength difference between green and red is greater.

    B. may be best explained by the double-opponent cells in the cortex.

    C. may be best explained by the single-opponent cells in the retina and LGN.

    D. both B and C.

5. The phenomenon of color constancy refers to the fact that

    A. the perceived color of an object never changes.

    B. the perceived color of an object is uniquely determined by the spectrum of the reflected light from the object.

    C. the perceived color of an object is relatively constant with respect to the changing lighting conditions.

    D. the perceived color of an object is independent of the colors of other objects around it.

■ *TRUE/FALSE QUESTIONS*
(If false, explain why)

1. All color vision systems have three types of cones with different spectral sensitivities. _____

2. The R cones are more sensitive to red light because the R pigment has a larger probability of absorbing long wavelength photons. _____

3. There are only two types of cones, the R and G types, in the fovea. _____

4. The amino acid sequence of the G pigment is closer to the B pigment than to the R pigment. _____

5. The R-center/G-surround single-opponent cells are best stimulated by red light in the center and green light in the surround of the receptive field. _____

6. The fact that we do not see reddish green or bluish yellow may be explained by either the single-opponent or double-opponent cells in the brain. _____

7. If two colored patches are indistinguishable by our eyes, the light spectral compositions from the two patches must be very similar. _____

■ SYNTHETIC QUESTIONS AND QUANTITATIVE PROBLEMS

1. Would we still have color vision if, instead of three types of cones, all cones were the same and each had all three types of visual pigments?

2. When red, green, and blue lights are projected together on a screen we see white light. When red, green, and blue paint pigments are mixed, however, the resulting color is black. Explain why.

3. The absorbance spectra of all three types of cone pigments are rather broad with large overlaps between them (see Figure 24–3 in the textbook, p. 456). This feature could either be an unimportant byproduct of the sloppiness of biological building blocks or it might have some functional significance. To gain some insight on this issue, consider a hypothetical visual system whose three types of cone pigments have the "perfect" absorbance spectra shown below. Would the system be able to discriminate, for example, a red light at 600 nm from a blue light at 430 nm?

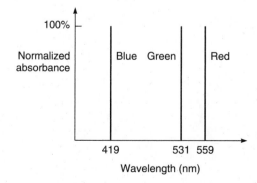

Figure 24–1

ANSWERS

◼ COMPLETION PROBLEMS

1. 400; 700.

2. primary colors; three.

3. opsin; retinal; opsin.

4. red-green; yellow-blue; white-black.

5. red; green.

6. X; seventh; third.

◼ MULTIPLE CHOICE QUESTIONS

1. D.

2. C.

3. D.

4. B.

5. C.

■ TRUE/FALSE QUESTIONS

1. False. Any system that can compare responses of at least *two* types of photoreceptors with different spectral sensitivity can have color vision.

2. True

3. True

4. False. G pigment sequence is closer to R pigment sequence.

5. False. They are best stimulated by a red spot in the center. R-center/G-surround double-opponent cells are best stimulated by red light in the center and green light in the surround.

6. True

7. False. Many lights with different spectral compositions can generate the same pattern of activity in the three types of cones, and thus appear to have the same color.

■ SYNTHETIC QUESTIONS AND QUANTITATIVE PROBLEMS

1. No. The three types of pigments would only generate a broad spectral response for all the hypothetical cones. There is no way to tell which proportion of a cone response is generated by which pigments.

2. Paint does not emit light but reflects light. It appears to have a certain color because it absorbs light with that color much less than light with other colors. When paints of different colors are mixed the resulting mixture will absorb light strongly at all wavelengths and will thus appear black.

3. No. Both colors would appear black to the system since there would be no absorption of light by cones in either case. The system could only distinguish stimuli with different proportions of light at 419, 531, and 559 nm. Everything else would appear black to the system.

25

Sensory Experience and the Formation of Visual Circuits

Overview

The connections between neurons in the brain are determined by both genetic programs and sensory experience. While the development of the overall structural organization of the brain is guided by molecular events, the establishment of fine patterns of connectivity in a mature brain depends on pre- and postnatal neural activities.

There is abundant evidence indicating that normal development of perception and the underlying neural circuits require sensory experience. Early sensory deprivation can cause irreversible deficiency in an animal's perceptual abilities, paralleled by the abnormal development of neural connections in the brain. Deprivation at later stages has much less effect. The synapses in the brain are constantly being tuned by sensory experience throughout life. This type of synaptic modification forms the basis of learning and memory.

The formation of ocular dominance columns in the primary visual cortex provides an ideal system for investigating the mechanism of activity-dependent neural plasticity. The two key elements involved are cooperation among nearby inputs from the same eyes and competition between the two different eyes. The cooperative process tends to stabilize nearby LGN projections from the same eye, thus generating the spatial extent of the columns. At the same time the competition between projections from the two eyes acts to separate LGN projections from the different eyes into non-overlapping regions.

These two processes are reflected at the cellular level. The Hebbian rule states that coincident activity in the pre- and postsynaptic elements of a synapse leads to the strengthening of that synapse. The synchronous activation of nearby LGN projections increases the probability of their firing the cortical cells that receive common inputs from these projections. This in turn increases the probability of synaptic enhancement for the synapses involved. On the other hand, projections from different eyes tend to fire more asynchronously. Consequently, when a cell in the cortex is driven by projections from one eye, the projections from the other eye are likely to be silent and will not be strengthened. As nearby projections from one eye to a cortical cell get stronger, the projections from the other eye to the same cortical cell becomes weaker.

The NMDA-type of glutamate receptors are believed to be responsible for the Hebbian type of synaptic modifications. Activation of this type of receptor requires simultaneous activity in the pre- and postsynaptic terminals. The resulting Ca^{2+} inflow through the activated receptor-channels triggers a second-messenger system that leads to synaptic modification.

Objectives

1. Understanding the influence of sensory experience on both behavior and neural circuits.

2. Understanding the concept of the critical periods in development.

3. Understanding how the ocular-dominance columns form in the primary visual cortex.

4. Understanding the Hebbian rule of synaptic plasticity and its implementation through the NMDA-type of glutamate receptors.

■ COMPLETION PROBLEMS

1. Ocular dominance columns are normally _____ in size for each eye. Early visual deprivation of the right eye will cause the right eye columns to _____.

2. As little as _____ week(s) of visual deprivation in the first _____ month(s) of life of a monkey will lead to a nearly complete loss of cortical responsiveness to stimulation of the deprived eye and a loss of vision in that eye. Comparable deprivation in an adult has _____ effect.

3. The retinal ganglion cells are spontaneously _____ *in utero*, independent of any visual information. Neighboring cells in the fetal retina tend to be active _____.

4. According to the Hebbian hypothesis, coincident activity in the pre- and postsynaptic elements of a synapse leads to the _____ of that synapse.

5. The binding of the transmitter _____ is not sufficient to activate the NMDA receptors because the ion channel of this receptor is normally blocked by _____. The block is removed by _____ of the cell membrane. The activated receptor-channel allows _____ to flow into the postsynaptic cell to trigger second-messenger systems.

■ MULTIPLE CHOICE QUESTIONS

1. The segregation of retinal inputs from the two eyes into different LGN layers

    A. does not depend on any neural activity.

    B. happens before birth.

    C. depends on activities caused by external visual stimulation.

    D. is genetically programmed through molecular recognition.

2. The formation of ocular dominance columns in the primary visual cortex

   A. requires synchronous activity in projections from the same eye and asynchronous activity in the projections from the two eyes.

   B. occurs before birth.

   C. is caused by spontaneous activity in the fetal retinas.

   D. is due to cooperation between projections from the two eyes.

■ *TRUE/FALSE QUESTIONS*
   (If false, explain why)

1. Synaptic plasticity cannot occur in a brain area after its critical period of development. _____

2. All neurons in the primary visual cortex have approximately the same critical period of development. _____

3. The segregation of inputs from each eye into different layers in the LGN does not depend on visual experience. _____

4. The NMDA receptors are normally activated by NMDA molecules in the brain. _____

5. The normal development of social behavior depends on the presence of specific environmental stimuli at specific stages of development. _____

SYNTHETIC QUESTIONS AND QUANTITATIVE PROBLEMS

1. There are about 10^{10} to 10^{11} neurons in the brain and each neuron makes about 10^3 to 10^4 synaptic contacts with other neurons. As a conservative estimation, assume that each synapse were either on or off, thus requiring only one bit of information to specify. How many bits of information would be required to specify all the neuronal connections in the brain? There are about 10^9 base pairs in the human DNA. Each pair can carry a maximum of two bits of information since there are four types of bases. If every base pair were coding nothing but synaptic connections, would the DNA carry enough information to specify all the synapses in the brain? Explain.

2. Describe the Hebbian rule of synaptic modification and discuss how the hypothesis is supported by the NMDA-type of glutamate receptors.

3. During the period of formation of the ocular-dominance columns in the normal primary visual cortex, what would happen if (1) there were only competition and not cooperation, or (2) there were only cooperation and not competition? Everything else is assumed to be normal.

ANSWERS

■ COMPLETION PROBLEMS

1. equal; shrink

2. one; six; no

3. active; synchronously

4. strengthening

5. glutamate; Mg^{2+}; depolarization; Ca^{2+}

■ MULTIPLE CHOICE QUESTIONS

1. B.

2. A.

▉ TRUE/FALSE QUESTIONS

1. False. Synaptic modification occurs throughout a brain's lifetime.

2. False. Different neurons can have different critical periods.

3. True

4. False. The NMDA receptors are normally activated by the neurotransmitter *glutamate* in the brain.

5. True

▉ SYNTHETIC QUESTIONS AND QUANTITATIVE PROBLEMS

1. About 10^{14} bits (or 10^7 megabytes of information) would be required to specify all the connections in the brain. For comparison, a modern personal computer typically has several megabytes of RAM memory and several hundreds of megabytes of hard disk space. The DNA would not carry enough information to specify all the synapses in the brain even if every base pair were coding synaptic connections.

2. The Hebbian rule states that coincident activity in the pre- and post-synaptic elements of a synapse leads to the strengthening of that synapse. Similarly, the activation of the NMDA-type of glutamate receptors requires simultaneous activation of the pre- and postsynaptic neurons. The presynaptic activity releases the neurotransmitter glutamate for binding to the receptor on the postsynaptic membrane. The depolarization of the postsynaptic neuron removes the Mg^{2+} block from the receptor channel to allow Ca^{2+} inflow upon the binding of glutamate. The increase of free Ca^{2+} concentration in the post-synaptic neuron is believed to cause synaptic modification through second-messenger systems.

3. (1) Without cooperation, cortical cells dominated by the same eyes would not stay together to form columns. The degree of eye dominance for each cell would also not be as strong as in the normal case. (2) Without competition there would be no ocular dominant cells in the cortex (except those occurring by chance) and the inputs from the two eyes would be more or less uniformly distributed across the cortex.

26

An Introduction to Movement

Overview

Motor processing begins with a neural representation of the movement—an image of the desired result. The study of the elementary components of these representations—what features of intended movements are coded in neural signs—is called motor psychophysics. The motor systems generate three types of movements: reflexes, rhythmic motor patterns, and voluntary movements. The motor structures of the central nervous system are organized as a hierarchical system with three levels of control: the spinal cord, the brain stem, and the motor areas of the cerebral cortex.

The spinal cord contains the motor neurons, which innervate skeletal muscles and represent the final common path of motor control. Within the ventral horn of the spinal cord, motor neurons are organized into motor neuron pools. Motor neurons that innervate axial muscles are located in medial regions of the ventral horn, whereas motor neurons that innervate distal limb muscles are located in lateral regions. The spinal cord also contains neuronal circuits that mediate reflexes and automatic behaviors.

The brain stem contains two parallel systems: medial descending pathways that play an important role in control of posture, and lateral descending pathways that play a role in controlling discrete goal-directed limb movements.

The highest level of motor control consists of the motor areas of cerebral cortex in the frontal lobe. These are essential for voluntary control of movement, especially fine movements of the fingers, and for coordinating and planning complex sequences of movements. A massive descending pathway, the corticospinal tract, projects from the motor areas of cortex to the spinal cord. This pathway has a large lateral component, the lateral corticospinal tract, which decussates in the lower medulla and projects to the lateral motor neurons in the spinal cord, and a smaller medial component, the ventral corticospinal tract, which does not decussate and projects to medial motor neurons. In humans and higher primates the fibers in the corticospinal tract make many direct connections to motor neurons. In more primitive mammals there are few such connections; in these animals the corticospinal tract primarily controls the flow of sensory information reaching higher levels of the brain.

In addition to the three hierarchical levels of control, there are two other important motor structures: the cerebellum and basal ganglia. These do not send pathways directly to the spinal cord. Instead, they act to regulate the main hierarchy of control, principally by their connections with the motor areas of the cortex.

A critical feature of the motor systems of the brain, most notably the primary motor area of the cortex, is that they have a somatotopic organization. Each area contains a motor map, in which movements of adjacent parts of the body are represented in adjacent areas of the brain.

Objectives

1. Understanding the main ideas of motor psychophysics and sensory psychophysics, especially with reference to the main attributes of sensation and movement.

2. Understanding the main types of movement.

3. Understanding the hierarchical system of motor control, including the three main levels of control, and their general functions.

4. Understanding what is meant by the motor neurons as the final common path.

5. Understanding the anatomical organization of motor neurons in the spinal cord and specifically the functions of medial and lateral motor neuron pools.

6. Understanding the functions of the important medial and lateral brain stem descending pathways.

7. Understanding the important motor areas of the cerebral cortex and the topographical organization of the primary motor cortex.

8. Understanding the origins and terminations of the two components of the corticospinal tract.

9. Understanding the role of the cerebellum and basal ganglia in motor control.

■ COMPLETION PROBLEMS

1. The principle that the same behavioral results can be carried out using different movement patterns is called _____.

2. A stereotyped response to a specific sensory stimulus is called a _____.

3. Agonist muscles, the prime movers in a particular action, are counter-balanced by _____ muscles.

4. The fibers of the corticospinal tract cross midline at the junction between the _____ and the spinal cord.

5. Corticospinal fibers control the motor neurons innervating trunk and limb muscles, whereas _____ fibers control the cranial nerve motor nuclei.

6. The main lateral descending pathway from the brain stem is the _____ tract.

7. The mechanical properties of the muscles, bones, and joints, which the motor systems must take into account in planning movement, are referred to collectively as the _____.

8. The term "final common path" refers to the _____.

■ MULTIPLE-CHOICE QUESTIONS

1. Motor neurons innervating individual limb muscles

    A. are clustered close together in aggregates typically confined to a single spinal segment.

    B. form discontinuous clusters located at several segments.

    C. form longitudinal aggregates frequently spanning 3 – 4 segments.

2. Axons that descend from the brain stem in the lateral columns of the spinal white matter are most likely to project to motor neurons innervating

    A. shoulder or pelvic girdle muscles.

    B. distal muscles.

    C. proximal muscles.

    D. extensor muscles.

3. Medial propriospinal neurons

    A. play an important role in coordinating hand and finger movements.

    B. receive inputs from the rubrospinal tract.

    C. make highly specific connections to only a few motor neuron pools.

    D. may project to motor neurons over many segments of the spinal cord.

4. Which descending system is principally responsible for coordinating head movements with visual input and eye movements?

    A. The corticospinal tract.

    B. The reticulospinal tract.

    C. The tectospinal tract.

    D. The rubrospinal tract.

5. Motor neurons innervating axial muscles are located in the

    A.   medial part of the ventral horn.

    B.   lateral part of the ventral horn.

    C.   medial part of the dorsal horn.

    D.   lateral part of the dorsal horn.

6. Which is *not* true of the lateral corticospinal system?

    A.   It decussates in the medullary pyramids.

    B.   Some of its axons terminate in the dorsal horn.

    C.   All of its axons synapse directly on motor neurons in the lateral part of the ventral horn.

    D.   Its axons originate from several areas of the cerebral cortex.

■ TRUE/FALSE QUESTIONS
(If false, explain why)

1. The motor neurons in the spinal cord are confined to the dorsal horn. _____

2. Descending fibers in the lateral columns tend to make widespread and diffuse connections within the spinal cord. _____

3. A lesion that selectively affected the lateral columns of the spinal cord would have the greatest impact on control of hand and finger movements. _____

4. All of the fibers in the corticospinal tract originate in the motor areas of the frontal lobe. _____

5. Neither the cerebellum nor the basal ganglia send axons directly to the spinal cord. _____

■ MATCHING PROBLEMS

1. Vestibulospinal tract

2. Reticulospinal tract

3. Tectospinal tract

4. Rubrospinal tract

5. Lateral corticospinal tract

6. Ventral corticospinal tract

A. coordination of head and eye movement

B. fine control of fingers

C. control of balance

D. maintenance of posture

E. cortical control of axial muscles

F. contribution to control of reaching and manipulating objects

■ SYNTHETIC QUESTIONS AND QUANTITATIVE PROBLEMS

1. Carry out the experiment illustrated in Figure 26–1 in the textbook (p. 490) by writing your name with a pen held in your right hand, left hand, teeth, and toes. Does the signature look the same in all cases? What features of the result stay the same? Provide a different example of motor equivalence.

2. Perform the following experiment. Draw two circles on a large piece of paper. The circles should have a diameter of 1 cm and be 10 cm apart. Place the paper in front of you. With a felt-tip pen, try to touch each circle alternately lightly. First carry out the experiment while counting slowly to 20 (about 1 touch per second). Now repeat the experiment (with a new piece of paper) while counting and touching the paper as fast as possible. Count the errors (number of touches outside a circle) made in each trial. Now repeat both the previous experiments, but with your eyes closed. Count the errors again. Graph or tabulate the

results. Pay particular attention to the effect of increased speed on accuracy. Does this effect change when the eyes are closed? What does this tell us about the role of vision in the speed-accuracy trade-off?

3. Describe a Jacksonian seizure. How does the nature of this seizure reveal something about how the motor areas of the brain are organized?

4. Characterize the movement disorders resulting from lesions to the cerebellum and basal ganglia. Why don't lesions of either of these areas produce paralysis? How would you characterize the general function of these areas?

5. Using specific references to the motor structures and pathways described in the textbook, give an example of (a) parallel organization in the motor systems, and (b) serial organization in the motor systems.

ANSWERS

◼ COMPLETION PROBLEMS

1. motor equivalence

2. reflex

3. antagonist

4. medulla

5. corticobulbar

6. rubrospinal

7. motor plant

8. motor neurons

◼ MULTIPLE-CHOICE QUESTIONS

1. C.

2. B.

3. D.

4. C.

5. A.

6. C.

TRUE/FALSE QUESTIONS

1. False. The motor neurons in the spinal cord are confined to the *ventral* horn.

2. False. Descending fibers in the lateral columns tend to make *specific and sharply focused* connections within the spinal cord.

3. True

4. False. Some of the fibers in the corticospinal tract originate in the motor areas of the frontal lobe, but others arise in the somatosensory areas of the parietal lobe.

5. True

MATCHING PROBLEMS

1. C.

2. D.

3. A.

4. F.

5. B.

6. E.

■ SYNTHETIC QUESTIONS AND QUANTITATIVE PROBLEMS

1. In general, the signatures will not be identical. They will vary especially in their size, accuracy, and smoothness. What remains the same is the form of the letters and the overall style of the signature. There are many examples of motor equivalence, in which the same behavioral result is achieved by different means. For example, one can eat a bowl of rice with a fork, spoon or chopsticks, using fingers alone, or even by bringing the bowl to the mouth and eating rice without using the fingers.

2. Individual results will vary in this experiment, but when many subjects are tested the results typically show that the number of errors increases with increasing speed when the eyes are open, but show little or no change when the eyes are closed. This indicates that the use of vision to guide movement is an important factor contributing to the speed-accuracy trade-off. Since processing visual information and using it to guide movement takes time, vision improves accuracy much more effectively when movements are slow.

3. A Jacksonian seizure typically begins as a series of involuntary contractions of a discrete part of the body, usually the fingers. The contractions gradually spread to more proximal parts of the arm, then the trunk and other muscles. Hughlings Jackson, the nineteenth century neurologist who first described this type of seizure, correctly surmised, on the basis of his observations alone, that the predictable order of spread revealed a somatotopic representation of body parts in the motor areas of cortex. Later physiological studies confirmed his theory.

4. Lesions of the cerebellum lead to impairments of motor coordination and movement accuracy. Lesions of the basal ganglia lead to loss of spontaneous movement, involuntary movements, and disturbances of posture. In neither case is there actual paralysis or even significant weakness. This is because neither structure projects directly to the spinal cord. Rather both structures exert their influence on movement by connections with other motor structures, especially the motor areas of the cerebral cortex. Therefore, the general function of these areas is not to initiate or directly control movement, but rather to regulate movement, to make it more accurate, smooth, and coordinated.

5. Parallel organization is clearly seen in the separate descending pathways to the spinal cord from the brain stem. For example, the reticulospinal, vestibulospinal, and tectospinal all project to medial motor neuron pools in the spinal cord, and each plays a different role in the generation and control of movement. An example of serial organization is the projection from the motor area of the cortex onto neurons in the reticular nuclei, which then project to the spinal cord.

27

Muscles and Their Receptors

Overview

The ultimate purpose of the elaborate neural processing by the motor systems of the brain is to control the contraction of skeletal muscle. To accomplish this, the nervous system monitors the state of the muscles. This proprioceptive information is provided by specialized receptors in muscles, especially muscle spindles and Golgi tendon organs.

The basic unit of motor function is the motor unit, which consists of a single motor neuron and all the muscle fibers that it innervates. The nervous system can grade the force of a contraction in two ways. First, it can vary the rate of firing of individual motor neurons, a mechanism called rate modulation. Second, the nervous system can vary the number of motor units active at any given time, a mechanism called recruitment. Based on their physiological and histochemical properties, muscle fibers (and their corresponding motor units) are classified as (1) slow fatigue-resistant, (2) fast fatigue-resistant, and (3) fast fatigable. When the nervous system recruits motor units to produce a specific amount of force, slow fatigue-resistant units are always recruited first, followed by fast fatigue-resistant units, and finally fast fatigable units. This fixed order of recruitment is based on the size of the motor neuron cell bodies and is thus referred to as the size principle.

Muscle spindles are encapsulated structures with specialized muscle fibers. They are innervated by both sensory and motor axons. Because of their parallel arrangement to skeletal muscle fibers, they signal changes in the length of muscles. Golgi tendon organs are encapsulated structures in which sensory endings are entwined among the braided collagen fibers at the junction between muscle fibers and tendons. Because they are arranged in series with muscle fibers, they signal changes in tension of muscles. Muscle spindles have two distinct types of receptors, primary and secondary endings. Both types of endings signal the steady-state length of muscles, but the primary ending also signals dynamic changes in muscle length. The motor axons innervating muscle spindles, termed gamma motor neurons, allow the nervous system to adjust their sensitivity. This is especially important when muscles shorten. Without activation of gamma motor neurons, muscle spindles would otherwise fall silent.

Objectives

1. Understanding the motor unit and its importance in motor control.

2. Understanding the two ways in which the nervous system grades the force of muscle contraction.

3. Understanding the size principle of motor unit recruitment.

4. Understanding the structure of muscle spindles and Golgi tendon organs.

5. Understanding the different types of information signaled by muscle spindles and Golgi tendon organs and how this functional difference arises from the anatomical arrangement of the two types of receptors.

6. Understanding dynamic and steady-state changes in muscle length and how muscle spindles signal these distinct types of information.

7. Understanding how motor innervation of muscle spindles is used to adjust the sensitivity of these sensory receptors and why this control is necessary.

COMPLETION PROBLEMS

1. Sensory input about the lengths of the muscles and the forces they generate is called _____ information.

2. In tetanus, the forces generated by individual muscle twitches _____, producing a larger total force than in a single twitch.

3. Muscle spindles are arranged in _____ with extrafusal muscle fibers. Therefore, they primarily detect muscle _____.

4. Tendon organs are arranged in _____ with extrafusal muscle fibers. Therefore, they primarily detect muscle _____.

5. When the intrafusal fibers of a muscle spindle are stretched, or "loaded," the sensory endings _____ their rate of firing. When the intrafusal fibers are unloaded, the rate of firing of the sensory endings _____.

6. Because of their high degree of sensitivity during the dynamic phase of movement, _____ endings of muscle spindles are very sensitive to small changes in muscle length.

MULTIPLE CHOICE QUESTIONS

1. The term "innervation ratio" refers to which of the following?

   A. The number of muscle fibers innervated by a motor neuron.

   B. The extent of the skin surface innervated by a dorsal root ganglion cell.

   C. The number of sensory receptors innervated by a dorsal root ganglion cell.

   D. The number of motor neurons innervating a muscle fiber.

2. Recruitment refers to the ability of the central nervous system to increase or decrease muscle tension by

   A. activating more or fewer of the muscle fibers within a motor unit.

   B. modulating the rate of firing of individual muscle fibers within a motor unit.

   C. activating more or fewer of the motor units within a motor neuron pool.

   D. modulating the rate of firing of individual motor units within a motor neuron pool.

3. The size principle of motor unit recruitment implies that

   A. higher motor centers can activate individual motor units in any order.

   B. on average, motor units with fast twitch contraction times will be used more often than those with slow twitch contraction times.

   C. low resistance exercises will strengthen all motor units equally.

   D. as the discharge rate of a motor neuron increases, more of the muscle fibers it innervates will contract.

   E. motor units that are most susceptible to fatigue will only fire in near-maximal contractions.

4. Which of the following will maximally increase the firing rate of a Ib afferent fiber?

   A. Electrical stimulation of gamma motor neurons.

   B. Electrical stimulation of Ia fibers.

   C. Electrical stimulation of alpha motor neurons.

5. The firing rate of primary endings of group Ia afferents is sensitive to

   A. changes in steady-state length of extrafusal fibers.

   B. the velocity of length change of extrafusal fibers.

   C. vibration of a muscle.

   D. sharp taps to a muscle tendon

   E. all of the above.

6. Contraction of an intrafusal muscle fiber by activation of gamma motor neurons

   A. increases the sensitivity of the muscle spindle.

   B. contributes significant force to a muscle contraction.

   C. increases the sensitivity of the Golgi tendon organ.

   D. decreases the discharge rate in spindle afferents.

7. If an alpha motor neuron is stimulated, causing the muscle it innervates to contract, but at the same time the gamma motor neurons to that muscle are not stimulated, which of the following would be expected?

   A. There would be no change in spindle afferent firing rate.

   B. There would be an increase in spindle afferent firing rate.

   C. There would be a decrease in spindle afferent firing rate.

■ *TRUE/FALSE QUESTIONS*
(If false, explain why)

1. The innervation ratio of motor units is lower for finger muscles than for muscles of the thigh. _____

2. Slow fatigue-resistant muscle fibers produce less tension than fast fatigable muscle fibers. _____

3. The muscle fibers innervated by a single motor neuron are all of the same type. _____

4. Both muscle spindles and Golgi tendon organs are encapsulated receptors with myelinated, large-diameter sensory axons. _____

5. The primary nerve endings of muscle spindles are sensitive only to the velocity of a stretch and not to steady-state muscle length. _____

6. In voluntary movements, the sensory endings of muscle spindles usually fall silent. _____

7. Gamma motor neurons control the sensitivity of Golgi tendon organs. _____

◼ MATCHING PROBLEMS

1. Alpha motor neuron

2. Gamma motor neuron

3. Primary spindle ending

4. Secondary spindle ending

5. Golgi tendon organ

A. dynamic and steady-state length receptor

B. tension receptor

C. controls sensitivity of spindle endings

D. controls force of muscle contraction

E. steady-state length receptor

◼ SYNTHETIC QUESTIONS AND QUANTITATIVE PROBLEMS

1. What is a motor unit? Explain why the motor unit has been referred to as the "quantal unit of motor function."

2. Define innervation ratio. Which muscles have large innervation ratios and which muscles small innervation ratios? Compare the concept of innervation ratio to the concept of receptive field in sensory systems. Are they analogous?

3. Identify and briefly explain the two mechanisms by which the nervous system modulates the force of muscle contraction. Compare these to the mechanisms by which sensory systems encode the intensity of a stimulus. Are they analogous?

4. Briefly describe the size principle of motor unit recruitment. Explain why this property of motor neurons simplifies the task of modulating muscle forces.

5. Distinguish between an unfused and a fused tetanus. If most muscle contractions involve an unfused tetanus in individual motor units, why does the overall muscle force appear smooth?

6. Make an outline of the three types of muscle fibers. For each type, characterize the physiological properties (speed of contraction, fatigability, and tension output).

7. Identify the three components of muscle spindles and the functional role of each.

8. Which receptor—muscle spindle or Golgi tendon organ—is better suited for sensing the effects of fatigue in muscles? Explain why.

9. Illustrate with a simple sketch how activation of gamma motor neurons can increase the sensitivity of spindle endings.

10. Explain what is meant by alpha-gamma coactivation. Why is such a mode of activation necessary? Can you think of a situation in which alpha-gamma coactivation would not be advantageous?

11. Consider the following phenomenon. When a vibrator is placed over the biceps muscle of a blindfolded subject, the subject experiences the illusion that the elbow joint is more extended than it really is. Explain why this error in position sense occurs. Identify the sensory receptor that is involved. What does this phenomenon tell us about the role of this receptor in conscious position sense?

ANSWERS

■ COMPLETION PROBLEMS

1. proprioceptive

2. summate

3. parallel; length

4. series; tension

5. increase; decreases

6. primary

■ MULTIPLE CHOICE QUESTIONS

1. A.

2. C.

3. E.

4. C.

5. E.

6. A.

7. C.

■ *TRUE/FALSE QUESTIONS*

1. True

2. True

3. True

4. True

5. False. The primary nerve endings of muscle spindles are sensitive both to the velocity of a stretch and also to steady-state muscle length.

6. False. In voluntary movements the sensory endings of muscle spindles usually maintain their firing because of alpha-gamma coactivation.

7. False. Gamma motor neurons control the sensitivity of *muscle spindles*.

■ *MATCHING PROBLEMS*

1. D.

2. C.

3. A.

4. E.

5. B.

■ SYNTHETIC QUESTIONS AND QUANTITATIVE PROBLEMS

1. The motor unit comprises a single motor neuron and all the muscle fibers it innervates. It is the quantal unit of motor function because it is the smallest unit that can be independently controlled by the nervous system. Individual muscle fibers cannot be independently controlled by the nervous system. All the muscle fibers making up a motor unit must contract as a unit.

2. Innervation ratio is the number of muscle fibers innervated by a single motor neuron. This ratio is low in muscles that carry out fine, discrete actions, such as finger and eye muscles. It is high in muscles that must exert forceful contractions, such as muscles of the trunk and legs. A sensory receptive field is the area on a receptive sheet which when stimulated causes a given receptor to respond. When receptive fields are small, the spatial precision of sensory will be high, just as motor units with a low innervation ratio allow greater precision of muscular control. Thus the concepts are indeed analogous.

3. The nervous system grades the force of a contraction by modulating the rate of firing in individual motor neurons (rate coding). This is analogous to a frequency code for stimulus intensity in which higher stimulus intensities are coded as higher firing rates. The nervous system can also increase the strength of a contraction by recruiting more motor neurons. This is analogous to the population code for stimulus intensity, in which higher stimulus intensities cause more sensory receptors to be activated.

4. Motor neurons are not recruited in any arbitrary order. Instead, the smallest motor neurons (whose motor units produce smaller forces, have slower contraction times, and show less tendency to fatigue) are always recruited before the larger motor neurons (whose motor units produce larger forces, have faster contraction times, and fatigue more quickly). This fixed order of recruitment is explained by the different cellular properties of small and large motor neurons. Thus, higher centers do not have to decide which motor neurons to activate first. The details of recruitment order are determined at the level of the motor neuron pool.

5. In a tetanus individual twitches occur so closely together in time that their forces summate, producing a greater amount of force than can be

produced in a single twitch. In an unfused tetanus the individual twitches can still be detected as ripples in the force produced by the motor unit. In a fused tetanus the twitches occur so closely together that they can no longer be distinguished and the motor unit's force appears smooth. Even when individual motor units are contracting with unfused tetanus, the overall force of the whole muscle appears smooth, because the firing of the different motor units is not synchronized. Therefore, the ripples occur at different times for each motor unit, and they tend to average out in the force of the whole muscle.

6.

Type	Speed of Contraction	Fatigability	Tension Output
Slow fatigue-resistant	Slow	Resistant to fatigue	Low
Fast fatigue-resistant	Fast	Resistant to fatigue	Intermediate
Fast fatigable	Fast	Fatigues quickly	High

7. Muscle spindles consist of three components: specialized muscle fibers, sensory endings, and motor endings. The specialized muscle fibers, termed intrafusal fibers, are attached in parallel with the ordinary skeletal muscle fibers. As the muscle is stretched, the intrafusal fibers also increase in length, thus providing a replica of the whole muscle. The sensory endings wrap around the intrafusal muscle fibers and increase their firing rate as the fibers are stretched, thus signaling changes in the length of the whole muscle. The motor endings innervate the ends of the intrafusal fibers and can cause them to contract. In this way they regulate the sensitivity of the muscle spindle.

8. Fatigue involves a reduction in muscle force, even as the level of activation remains the same. The Golgi tendon organ, since it senses the force produced by a muscle, is better suited to sensing the effects of fatigue. Nevertheless, the nervous system must also take into account signals from muscle spindles. This is because the force might be decreasing not because of fatigue, but because the muscle length is changing (force also depends on muscle length). Thus, monitoring input from both receptors is necessary to sense the effects of fatigue.

9. Activation of gamma motor neurons causes contraction and shortening of the end regions of intrafusal fibers, thus loading the spindle and making it more responsive to stretches (see Figure 27–9 in the textbook, p. 511, as a model for a sketch).

10. Alpha-gamma activation is the simultaneous activation of alpha motor neurons and gamma motor neurons in a voluntary movement. This is necessary to prevent the spindle from slackening while the muscle is shortening, which would make it unresponsive to small unexpected changes in length. In some movements a muscle contracts while the muscle is lengthening. For example, if you bend your knees slowly to lower your body to the floor, the extensor muscles of the knee will contract continuously in order to prevent flexion from occurring too rapidly. In such a "lengthening contraction" there is no need to activate gamma motor neurons since the spindle will not slacken. In fact, activating the gamma motor neurons might cause the spindle firing to saturate. Therefore, it is advantageous to have independent control of alpha and gamma motor neurons, as all mammals do.

11. Vibration is a very potent stimulus for the primary endings of muscle spindles, since it applies a repetitive phasic change of length. Vibration causes the muscle spindles in the biceps muscle to fire at a high rate, even though the net length of the muscle does not change. The nervous system interprets this as an actual change of length of the muscle. This phenomenon indicates that the information received by muscle spindles reaches conscious perception and that it probably plays an important role in position sense.

28

Spinal Reflexes

Overview

Motor coordination is the process of linking together the contractions of independent muscles so that they act together. The most elementary form of coordination is the reflex, a stereotyped response to a specific sensory stimulus. Spinal reflexes are those in which the essential neural circuitry is entirely contained within the spinal cord. The monosynaptic stretch reflex provides a simple model of reflex action. Afferent fibers from muscle spindles make excitatory connections with motor neurons that innervate the same muscle as well as muscles having a similar action. They also make inhibitory connections, through an interneuron, with motor neurons that innervate opposing muscles. The stretch reflex circuits produce resistance to a quick stretch of the muscle and are therefore important in regulating muscle tone. Afferent fibers from Golgi tendon organs inhibit, through an interneuron, motor neurons that innervate the same muscles from which the afferents arise. This circuit is important for regulating muscle force.

Many spinal reflexes are triggered by stimulation of the skin. In flexion withdrawal reflexes a nociceptive input excites, through polysynaptic pathways, motor neurons that innervate flexor muscles of the limb from which the afferents arise. In addition, the same input both inhibits motor neurons that innervate opposing muscles and excites extensor muscles in the opposite limb. The scratch reflex, observed in furry animals, is noteworthy in that it produces rhythmic alternating muscle contractions, without rhythmic stimulation. This provides an example of how spinal circuits are capable of producing sustained patterns of rhythmic output.

Spinal circuits are also capable of generating the rhythmic patterns of muscle contractions used in walking. These circuits have been studied in spinal cats, experimental animals in which the spinal cord is transected to isolate the part of the spinal cord that controls the hind limbs from control by the brain. Such animals exhibit a near normal walking pattern on a moving treadmill, but they do need external support for balance. In normal cats, pathways from the brain stem activate locomotion and control balance. Pathways from the cerebral cortex are necessary to adapt locomotion to the environment.

Objectives

1. Understanding the characteristics of spinal reflexes and their importance in motor coordination.

2. Understanding the neural circuitry of the stretch, flexion withdrawal, and scratch reflexes.

3. Understanding the functional importance of the stretch reflex.

4. Understanding the connections of the inhibitory interneurons of the spinal cord that receive input from muscle spindles and Golgi tendon organs.

5. Understanding the experimental evidence that locomotion in mammals is largely controlled by spinal circuits, and the role of supraspinal structures in the control of walking.

■ *COMPLETION PROBLEMS*

1. The circuitry of the stretch reflex acts as a negative _____ loop to resist changes in muscle length.

2. The stretch reflex produces a brisk but short-lasting _____ contraction, triggered by the change in muscle length, and a weaker but longer-lasting _____ contraction, determined by the static stretch of muscles at the new length.

3. The stretch reflex is referred to as _____ because there is only a single synapse between the afferent neuron and the motor neuron.

4. The Ib inhibitory interneuron receives input from three types of receptors: Golgi tendon organs, _____ receptors, and _____ receptors.

5. The flexion-withdrawal reflex is associated with a crossed _____ response in the opposite limb.

6. Spinal circuits that coordinate rhythmic stepping patterns are referred to as _____ generators.

7. In _____ animals, spinal reflexes are heightened and stereotyped, making it easier to study the factors that control these reflexes.

8. The fixed spatial relationship between the location of a stimulus and the particular muscles that contract is called _____.

■ MULTIPLE CHOICE QUESTIONS

1. Stimulation of Ia afferents of muscle spindles by a quick stretch of a muscle leads to

A. excitation of both synergist and antagonist motor neurons.

B. inhibition of both synergist and antagonist motor neurons.

C. excitation of synergist motor neurons and inhibition of antagonist motor neurons.

D. inhibition of synergist motor neurons and excitation of antagonist motor neurons.

2. Which of the following responses is produced by a sharp tap of the biceps tendon of the arm?

   A.   Excitation of biceps motor neurons.

   B.   Inhibition of triceps motor neurons.

   C.   Inhibition of motor neurons innervating other elbow flexors.

   D.   A and B.

   E.   A, B, and C.

3. Reciprocal innervation in stretch reflexes results from

   A.   polysynaptic excitation by Ia afferents of antagonist motor neurons.

   B.   an interposed inhibitory neuron between Ia afferents and antagonist motor neurons.

   C.   monosynaptic inhibition by Ia afferents of antagonist motor neurons.

   D.   increased gamma firing to spindles in antagonist motor neurons.

4. Hyperactive stretch reflexes and spasticity can result from

   A.   peripheral nerve disease.

   B.   motor neuron disease.

   C.   muscle disease.

   D.   disruption of central descending pathways.

   E.   all of the above.

5. The group Ib inhibitory interneuron in the spinal cord receives input from

   A.   cutaneous receptors.

   B.   joint receptors.

   C.   Golgi tendon organs.

   D.   all of the above.

6. A painful stimulus applied to the right foot leads to

    A. monosynaptic excitation of motor neurons innervating flexor muscles of the right leg.

    B. polysynaptic excitation of motor neurons innervating extensor muscles of the left leg.

    C. polysynaptic inhibition of motor neurons innervating flexor muscles of the left leg.

    D. polysynaptic inhibition of motor neurons innervating extensor muscles of the right leg.

7. Flexion-withdrawal reflexes

    A. are absent in animals with transection of the spinal cord.

    B. are monosynaptic reflexes.

    C. include reciprocal inhibition of ipsilateral extensor motor neurons.

    D. all of the above.

    E. none of the above.

8. Locomotion in cats is still possible following

    A. transection of the brain stem at the level of the midbrain.

    B. transection of the spinal cord.

    C. transection of the dorsal roots.

    D. all of the above.

9. Central pattern generators for locomotion are networks of neurons that generate rhythmic alternating activity in flexor and extensor muscles. These networks are located in the

    A. spinal cord.

    B. brain stem.

    C. cerebellum.

    D. motor cortex.

◼ TRUE/FALSE QUESTIONS
(If false, explain why)

1. Each Ia afferent makes excitatory connections with all the motor neurons innervating the same (homonymous) muscle. _____

2. Hypoactive stretch reflexes always result from lesions of the peripheral nerves or muscle. _____

3. Most reflex pathways are monosynaptic, like the stretch reflex. _____

4. Ia afferent axons make direct inhibitory synapses with motor neurons that innervate antagonist muscles. _____

5. A cutaneous stimulus on the sole of the foot always causes the same response, regardless of its intensity and quality. _____

6. When the dorsal roots carrying sensory input from a hind limb are cut, that limb will no longer participate in the scratch reflex. _____

7. Spinal circuits are only capable of producing gross flexion and extension of the limbs in walking; the fine details of the locomotor patterns require descending commands from higher centers. _____

◼ SYNTHETIC QUESTIONS AND QUANTITATIVE PROBLEMS

1. Define the two features of a stimulus that shape a reflex response. Choose one of the reflexes described in this chapter and describe specifically how these two features shape the reflex.

2. Define reciprocal innervation. Besides the stretch reflex, what other reflex exhibits reciprocal innervation. Of what importance is recipro-

cal innervation in voluntary movement? Describe how descending pathways make use of reflex circuits to produce reciprocal innervation.

3. Define muscle tone. Identify three functions of normal muscle tone.

4. Identify the three main levels of control that govern spinal reflexes. Give an example of each.

5. Explain what is meant by co-contraction. What function does it serve? How can the same circuits responsible for reciprocal innervation be used to accomplish co-contraction?

6. What is meant by active touch? What is the role of the Ib inhibitory interneuron in the control of active touch?

7. Make a sketch of the half-center model. Explain how this type of circuit can sustain alternating activity in opposing muscles without rhythmic input.

ANSWERS

▰ COMPLETION PROBLEMS

1. feedback

2. phasic; tonic

3. monosynaptic

4. joint; cutaneous

5. extension

6. central pattern

7. decerebrate

8. local sign

▰ MULTIPLE CHOICE QUESTIONS

1. C.

2. D.

3. B.

4. D.

5. D.

6. B.

7. C.

8. D.

9. A.

■ *TRUE/FALSE QUESTIONS*

1. True

2. False. Hypoactive stretch reflexes may also result from central lesions.

3. False. Most reflex pathways are polysynaptic. The stretch reflex is the only known example of a monosynaptic reflex in the mammalian nervous system.

4. False. Ia afferent axons make indirect inhibitory connections with motor neurons that innervate antagonist muscles, through an interposed interneuron.

5. False. A cutaneous stimulus on the sole of the foot always causes different reflex responses, depending on its quality and intensity.

6. False. When the dorsal roots carrying sensory input from a hind limb are cut, that limb will still produce a scratch reflex.

7. False. Spinal circuits produce a differentially timed and spatially distributed locomotor synergy.

■ SYNTHETIC QUESTIONS AND QUANTITATIVE PROBLEMS

1. Two features of a stimulus that are especially important in shaping a reflex response are the locus of the stimulus on the body and the strength of the stimulus. A good example of how these two features shape a reflex is seen in the scratch reflex. An irritative stimulus is applied to the flank of a furry animal. The location of the stimulus will affect which muscles contract to bring the paw to the precise location of the stimulus. The intensity of the stimulus will determine the magnitude of the movement, its duration, and latency.

2. Reciprocal innervation is the feature of reflex circuits that produces excitation of motor neurons innervating one muscle or group of muscles while at the same time producing inhibition of motor neurons that innervate opposing (antagonist) muscles. Most reflex circuits include reciprocal innervation. A good example is the flexion withdrawal reflex, in which a painful stimulus causes contraction of flexor muscles in a limb along with simultaneous relaxation (due to inhibition) of extensor muscles in the same limb. Reciprocal innervation is also important in voluntary movement; it is usually advantageous to relax antagonist muscles during movement so that the muscles responsible for the movement are not working against active muscle contraction. To accomplish this, the axons in many descending pathways send collateral axons to the Ia inhibitory neuron, so that inhibition of opposing muscles occurs automatically. Thus, higher centers do not have to send signals to each group of muscles.

3. Muscle tone is the force with which a muscle resists being lengthened. Muscle tone is important for postural control, by resisting swaying of the body. It also provides a mechanism for storing energy in muscles, like energy storage in springs, thus assisting in conserving energy. Finally, muscle tone smoothes movements, since it dampens sudden starts and stops.

4. The three levels of control of spinal reflexes are (1) individual muscles, (2) the muscles around a joint, and (3) the muscles of an entire limb. An example of individual muscle control is the monosynaptic stretch reflex. An example of control of the muscles at a joint is reciprocal innervation in the stretch reflex. An example of control of an entire limb is the flexion-withdrawal reflex.

5. Co-contraction is a mode of muscle activation in which opposing muscles increase their degree of contraction in parallel instead of in the normal reciprocal mode. Co-contraction is used to increase the stiffness around a joint in order to maximize stability or precision. The same circuits that are responsible for reciprocal innervation can achieve co-contraction because the inhibitory interneurons receive separate excitatory and inhibitory inputs from higher centers. By inhibiting the inhibitory interneurons, higher centers can change a reciprocal contraction to co-contraction.

6. Active touch refers to the use of fine exploratory movements of the fingers around or on the surface of an object. In active touch the control of the movements depends on information from cutaneous receptors concerning the tactile features of the surface, from Golgi tendon organs about how much force the muscles are exerting, and from joint receptors and other muscle receptors about the current positions of the fingers. All of these inputs converge on the Ib inhibitory interneuron, which inhibits motor neurons. The Ib inhibitory interneuron integrates the different types of information to modulate the muscle force and especially to prevent it from becoming too forceful when the fingers are touching the object.

7. The half-center model is illustrated in Figure 28–6 in the textbook (p. 524). This type of circuit provides sustained alternating activity in opposing muscles as long as there is a tonic excitation of each "half-center." This happens because the two half-centers inhibit each other. It is assumed that one half-center will initially fire more strongly than the other, perhaps because of random fluctuations in membrane excitability. When this happens the more active half-center will inhibit the other half-center, turning it off. Over time, however, the inhibition will fatigue or adapt and therefore lessen in intensity. As a result, the other half-center will begin to fire and this in turn will inhibit the half-center that was initially more active. This process will continue to cycle for as long as there is tonic excitation of the entire circuit. Thus, this type of circuit produces rhythmical output without rhythmical input.

29

Voluntary Movement

Overview

Planning for voluntary movement, as well as shaping it to the changing features of the environment, is accomplished by the higher motor centers of the brain: the motor areas of the cerebral cortex, the basal ganglia, and the cerebellum. The motor areas of the cerebral cortex are in the frontal lobe and consist of the primary motor cortex and the premotor areas. The primary motor cortex contains a precise somatotopic map of the body. In this region neurons fire in advance of movement and encode the force and direction of intended movements. They also receive information from somatosensory receptors about the consequences of movements. The premotor cortical areas include the supplementary motor cortex and the premotor cortex; these areas play a major role in the planning of goal-directed movements.

Both the cerebellum and the basal ganglia regulate movement indirectly. Neither structure sends its output directly to the spinal cord. Instead, both structures exert their influence on motor areas of the cerebral cortex and brain stem nuclei. The cerebellum acts as a comparator, compensating for errors by comparing intended movement with actual performance. It is also important for motor learning. The cerebellum consists of three functional divisions; the vestibulocerebellum, which governs eye movements and postural control; the spinocerebellum, which plays a major role in controlling the ongoing execution of movement; and the cerebrocerebellum, which assists the motor areas of the cortex in the planning and initiation of movement. Lesions of the cerebellum do not produce paralysis or weakness; instead, they lead to disorders of movement accuracy and coordination.

The basal ganglia consist of five interconnected nuclei deep within the cerebral hemispheres. Together they receive information from diverse areas of cerebral cortex, process that information, and send back signals to the same areas of cortex by way of the thalamus. The result of this processing is to assist in the planning and initiation of complex self-initiated movements. Lesions of the basal ganglia lead to involuntary movements, tremor, slowness of movement, and difficulty in initiating movement. An important disease involving the basal ganglia is Parkinson's disease, in which dopaminergic cells in the substantia nigra degenerate. The effects of this disease can be ameliorated, though not cured, by administering L-DOPA, a precursor of dopamine. This was one of the first neurological diseases to be successfully treated through pharmacologic intervention.

Objectives

1. Understanding the organization of the motor areas of the cerebral cortex.

2. Understanding the major experiments that elucidate the roles of the different cortical motor areas in controlling movement.

3. Understanding the major subdivisions of the cerebellum and their different roles in motor control, and the major deficits that result from lesions to the cerebellum.

4. Understanding the principal circuit of the cerebellum and how it functions as a comparator as well as in motor learning.

5. Understanding the overall anatomical organization of the basal ganglia, including the input nuclei, the intrinsic nuclei, and the output nuclei, and the role of the basal ganglia in movement control.

6. Understanding the pathophysiology and treatment of Parkinson's disease.

■ *COMPLETION PROBLEMS*

1. Lesions of the premotor cortical areas cause symptoms of _____, in which there is an inability to perform complex sequences or planned strategies.

2. The side loop through the cerebellar cortex ultimately has an _____ effect on the cells in the deep cerebellar nuclei.

3. The principal output neuron of the cerebellar cortex is the _____ cell.

4. The disorders of movement that result from cerebellar lesions are collectively referred to as _____.

5. The firing pattern of single neurons in primary motor cortex encodes the _____ of muscle contraction. The firing pattern of populations of neurons in primary motor cortex encodes the _____ of movement.

6. The cerebellar cortex receives its input through two types of neurons: _____ fibers and _____ fibers.

7. The caudate nucleus and putamen, though anatomically separate, consist of identical cell types and are together referred to as the _____.

■ *MULTIPLE CHOICE QUESTIONS*

1. A key difference between the patterns of discharge of neurons in the primary and supplementary motor cortex is that

    A. the supplementary motor cortex fires in advance of limb movement.

    B. many primary motor cortex neurons fire during both ipsilateral and contralateral movement.

    C. many supplementary motor cortex neurons fire specifically during simultaneous movements of both limbs.

    D. supplementary motor cortex neurons fire in advance of movements of the neck and trunk whereas primary motor cortex neurons fire only during limb and face movements.

2. Research indicates that when a subject mentally rehearses a complex sequence of finger movements, increased neural activity is found in the

    A. primary motor cortex.

    B. supplementary motor area.

    C. primary somatosensory cortex.

    D. cerebellum.

3. The premotor areas of the frontal lobe differ from the primary motor area in that

    A. muscle contractions are more easily stimulated with electrical currents in the primary motor cortex.

    B. only the primary motor cortex is somatotopically organized.

    C. the premotor cortex is more concerned with control of distal muscles than is the primary motor cortex.

    D. all of the above.

4. The most powerful excitation of Purkinje cells is produced by

   A. mossy fibers.

   B. parallel fibers.

   C. basket cells.

   D. climbing fibers.

5. The cortex of the lateral cerebellar hemispheres is most involved in

   A. movement planning.

   B. corrections to ongoing movements.

   C. modulation of the vestibular-ocular reflex.

6. The neurotransmitter typically most reduced in patients with Parkinson's disease is

   A. dopamine.

   B. norepinephrine.

   C. serotonin.

   D. acetylcholine.

7. A major output from the internal portion of the globus pallidus goes to the

   A. thalamus.

   B. spinal cord.

   C. cortex.

   D. cerebellum.

8. The substance actively transported across the blood-brain barrier is

   A. dopamine.

   B. L-DOPA.

   C. serotonin.

   D. gABA.

9. The primary output pathway of the basal ganglia goes to

   A.   the thalamus, then to the motor areas of the cortex.

   B.   the motor cortex directly, bypassing the thalamus.

   C.   the spinal cord.

   D.   the cerebellum.

10. The principal input nuclei of the basal ganglia are the

    A.   caudate and globus pallidus.

    B.   putamen and substantia nigra.

    C.   caudate and putamen.

    D.   globus pallidus and substantia nigra.

11. Which of the following is *not* a typical symptom of Parkinson's disease?

    A.   Tremor at rest.

    B.   Rigidity.

    C.   Weakness.

    D.   Slowness of movement.

■ TRUE/FALSE QUESTIONS
(If false, explain why)

1. Neurons in the primary motor cortex are activated when a subject mentally rehearses a voluntary movement.   _____

2. Electrical stimulation of the cerebral cortex evokes muscle contractions at the lowest intensity when the stimulating electrode is placed in the primary motor area.   _____

3. The cell bodies of Purkinje cells are found within the deep cerebellar nuclei.   _____

4. Dysmetria is a typical symptom of Parkinson's disease. _____

5. The basal ganglia sends its projecting axons to the spinal cord. _____

6. Parkinson's disease can be cured by administration of L-DOPA. _____

7. During visually guided tracking tasks, neurons in the basal ganglia fire later than cells in the cortical motor areas. _____

▦ MATCHING PROBLEMS

1. Primary motor area of cerebral cortex

2. Premotor cortex

3. Supplementary motor cortex

4. Vestibulocerebellum

5. Spinocerebellum

6. Cerebrocerebellum

7. Dentate, interposed, and fastigial nuclei

8. Caudate nucleus and putamen

9. Globus pallidus (internal segment) and substantia nigra (pars reticulata)

10. Substantia nigra

A. input nuclei of basal ganglia

B. receive synaptic input from Purkinje cells

C. contains neurons that encode direction and force of intended movements

D. contains neurons that synthesize dopamine

E. output nuclei of basal ganglia

F. governs eye movements and equilibrium

G. regulates ongoing movement

H. coordinates bilateral movements

I. assists in planning and initiation of movement

J. contains neurons whose activity is set-related

◼ SYNTHETIC QUESTIONS AND QUANTITATIVE PROBLEMS

1. Describe the experiment used to determine that the firing of single cells in the primary motor cortex is better related to muscle force than joint displacement.

2. Explain what is meant by the finding that cells in the primary motor cortex have broad tuning curves for movement direction. Explain why movement direction can be coded precisely despite this property of single cells.

3. Describe the similarities and differences between activation of the primary motor cortex and the supplementary motor area during (a) simple finger flexion-extension, (b) performance of a sequence of finger movements, and (c) mental rehearsal of a sequence of finger movements. What do these findings imply about the respective roles of the two structures?

4. Explain what is meant by the term "set-related neurons." Where have such neurons been found? Briefly describe the experimental approach used to discover such neurons.

5. Both the basal ganglia and the cerebellum form internal circuits or loops. Identify the key differences between these circuits (sources of input and targets of output). What implications do these differences have for the respective roles of these structures in movement control?

6. Identify the three subdivisions of the cerebellum, the anatomical area of the cerebellum that makes up each subdivision, the source of afferent input to that area, the deep nuclei to which that area projects, and the principal function.

7. Which component of the cerebellar circuit is considered to be most important for motor learning? Identify the types of motor learning in which the cerebellum has been shown to be important.

8. List the major nuclei of the basal ganglia. Identify whether each nucleus receives *input* from other structures, sends *output* to other structures, or performs *internal* processing.

9. Compare the major symptoms of Parkinson's disease to the major symptoms of cerebellar disease. Identify key differences and similarities. What do these symptoms tell us about the similarities and differences in the role of the basal ganglia and cerebellum in the control of movement?

ANSWERS

COMPLETION PROBLEMS

1. apraxia

2. inhibitory

3. Purkinje

4. ataxia

5. force; direction

6. climbing; mossy

7. neostriatum

MULTIPLE CHOICE QUESTIONS

1. C.

2. B.

3. A.

4. D.

5. A.

6. A.

7. A.

8. B.

9. A.

10. C.

11. C.

▄▄ *TRUE/FALSE QUESTIONS*

1. False. Neurons in the *supplementary motor area* are activated when a subject mentally rehearses a voluntary movement.

2. True

3. False. The cell bodies of Purkinje cells are found within the *cerebellar cortex*.

4. False. Dysmetria is a typical symptom of *cerebellar* disease.

5. False. The basal ganglia sends no projecting axons to the spinal cord. Its principal projection is to the cerebral cortex via the thalamus.

6. False. Only the *symptoms* of Parkinson's disease can be treated by administration of L-DOPA. A cure has not yet been discovered.

7. True

MATCHING PROBLEMS

1. C.

2. J.

3. H.

4. F.

5. G.

6. I.

7. B.

8. A.

9. E.

10. D.

SYNTHETIC QUESTIONS AND QUANTITATIVE PROBLEMS

1. While recording from a corticospinal tract neuron in the motor cortex of an awake monkey, the monkey was required to make flexion movements with two different loads: (a) a load opposing flexion, and (b) a load assisting flexion. The neuron fired only when the load opposed flexion and was silent when the load assisted flexion. Because the direction of movement was the same in both cases, the neuron's firing encodes force and not direction of movement.

2. The firing rate in individual neurons is recorded while a monkey moves its hand in different directions. The neuron fires for a broad range of movement direction, but its firing rate varies for different directions. Thus, it is "broadly tuned" for direction. Precise movement direction is coded by the combined output of many neurons.

3. During simple finger flexion only the primary motor cortex is activated. During performance of a sequence of finger movements both areas are activated. During mental rehearsal of the sequence only the supplementary motor area is activated. This finding implies that the motor cortex is involved in the execution of all voluntary finger movements, whereas the supplementary motor area is involved in planning sequences of movements.

4. Set-related neurons are those neurons whose activity is associated with the preparation to act. Set-related neurons have been found in the premotor cortex. The experimental approach used to discover such neurons involves recording from a neuron during a delay period between an instruction to make a specific movement and the onset of the movement.

5. Both the basal ganglia and the cerebellum receive inputs from the cerebral cortex. However, whereas the cerebellum also receives precisely organized information directly from sensory receptors, the basal ganglia do not. Both the basal ganglia and the cerebellum send outputs to the cerebral cortex, but the cerebellum also regulates movements through connections to brain stem nuclei. These differences reflect a difference in the roles of the two structures. The cerebellum plays a greater role in regulating the execution of ongoing movement, while the basal ganglia are more concerned with planning of movement.

6.

Subdivision	Area of cerebellum	Input	Output	Function
Vestibulo-cerebellum	Flocculo-nodular lobe	Vestibular nuclei	Vestibular nuclei	Eye move-ments and balance
Spino-cerebellum	Vermis and intermediate part of hemi-sphere	Spinal cord	Medial and lateral descending systems	Regulating ongoing exe-cution of movement
Cerebro-cerebellum	Lateral part of hemisphere	Cerebral cortex via pontine nuclei	Motor and premotor cortex	Planning and initiation of movement

7. The input to Purkinje cells from climbing fibers is considered to be the most important mechanism underlying motor learning. This input is capable of producing long-lasting changes in the efficacy of parallel fiber inputs to the Purkinje cells. Experiments have demonstrated a role for the cerebellum in adapting the vestibuloocular reflex when subjects wear reversing prisms. Another type of motor learning dependent on the cerebellum is the adjustment to new loads opposing arm movements.

8.

Nucleus	Function
Caudate nucleus	Input
Putamen	Input
Globus pallidus	
external segment	Intrinsic
Internal segment	Output
Subthalamic nucleus	Intrinsic
Substantia nigra	
Pars reticulata	Output
Pars compacta	Intrinsic

9. The major symptoms of Parkinson's disease include tremor, slowness of movement, lack of spontaneous movement, and rigidity. The major symptoms of cerebellar disease include delay in initiating movement, errors in range, force, rate, and regularity of movement. Lesions of neither structure produces paralysis or significant weakness. Therefore, both structures are important for regulating the quality of movement but are not necessary for directly initiating it. The main difference between the two structures is that lesions of the cerebellum more directly affect the ongoing execution of movement, while lesions of the basal ganglia interfere with the ability to correctly incorporate different movements into a motor act.

30

Genes and Behavior

Overview

Behavior is shaped by the interaction of genes with the environment. Genes direct the manufacture of proteins that are important in the formation of neural circuits that in turn underlie behavior. Thus, the relation of genes to behavior is generally indirect. Nonetheless, studies of identical twins separated early in life indicate that even complex behavioral traits like personality have a genetic component. Single genes are critically important for some simple traits, such as color vision or Huntington's disease.

More complex traits, such as schizophrenia or bipolar affective disorder, are controlled by many genes acting in concert.

New techniques for the introduction of specific mutations into the genes of flies or mice now permit experimental tests of the genetic control of specific behaviors. Such experiments have identified proteins that play a critical role in behaviors such as courtship and circadian rhythms in flies and other animals.

Objectives

1. Understanding in general the relationship between genes and behavior.

2. Understanding how studies of identical twins support the conclusion that there is a genetic component for personality, schizophrenia, and bipolar affective disorder.

3. Understanding sex chromosomes and how they relate to red-green color blindness.

4. Understanding the major symptoms of Huntington's disease and how the gene for it was located.

5. Understanding in general the techniques for creating mutant flies or mice with mutations in specific genes and what these techniques have revealed about molecules critical for courtship behavior and circadian rhythms in flies.

■ *COMPLETION PROBLEMS*

1. Darwin first postulated that variations in behavior are due in part to _____.

2. A mutation in which the sequence change is expressed even if only one of the two alleles of the gene is mutant is called _____.

3. Sequence variation in a gene is called _____.

4. Behavioral traits that are controlled by many genes are called _____.

5. A programmed series of stereotyped behaviors that an animal is capable of performing without prior experience is called a _____.

MULTIPLE CHOICE QUESTIONS

1. The relationship between genes and behavior is being studied extensively in

   A. *Caernorhabditis elegans*.

   B. *Drosophila*.

   C. mice.

   D. humans.

   E. all of the above

2. A single gene is critically important for

   A. sensitization in the blowfly.

   B. pointing in dogs.

   C. schizophrenia.

   D. bipolar affective disorder.

   E. all of the above.

3. Huntington's disease is characterized by

   A. heritability.

   B. chorea.

   C. dementia.

   D. onset late in life.

   E. all of the above.

4. The product of the *fruitless* gene in *Drosophila* is

   A. a metabolic protein.

   B. a nuclear protein.

   C. a structural protein.

   D. critical for the development of male-specific cells.

   E. critical for the development of female-specific cells.

5. The product of the *per* gene in *Drosophila* is

   A. a metabolic protein.

   B. a nuclear protein.

   C. a structural protein.

   D. critical for the development of male-specific cells.

   E. critical for the development of female-specific cells.

■ TRUE/FALSE QUESTIONS
(If false, explain why)

1. Identical twins separated early in life work in the same profession more often than would be expected by chance. _____

2. A mutation of a single gene is responsible for Huntington's disease. _____

3. A mutation of a single gene is responsible for schizophrenia. _____

4. Analysis of mosaic flies indicates that male courtship behavior requires that the entire brain be "male." _____

5. The product of the *per* gene in *Drosophila* feeds back to inhibit transcription of the gene. _____

■ MATCHING PROBLEMS

1. Circadian rhythms   A. chromosome 4

2. Color blindness   B. *fruitless* gene

3. Courtship behavior   C. *per* gene

4. Huntington's disease   D. polygenic

5. Schizophrenia   E. X chromosome

■ SYNTHETIC QUESTIONS AND QUANTITATIVE PROBLEMS

1. Describe in general terms the genetic basis of heritable behavior.

2. Explain how studies of relatives have shown that there is a genetic component to schizophrenia.

3. Explain what X-linked chromosomes are and how they relate to familial patterns of red-green color blindness in humans.

4. Describe how the gene for Huntington's disease was located.

5. Describe in general terms the technique for creating mice with mutations in a specific gene.

ANSWERS

◼ COMPLETION PROBLEMS

1. natural selection

2. dominant

3. polymorphism

4. polygenic

5. fixed-action pattern

◼ TRUE/FALSE QUESTIONS

1. True

2. True

3. False. Schizophrenia is polygenic.

4. False. Only certain parts of the brain need to be "male."

5. True

■ *MULTIPLE CHOICE QUESTIONS*

1. E.

2. A.

3. E.

4. D.

5. B.

■ *MATCHING PROBLEMS*

1. C.

2. E.

3. B.

4. A.

5. D.

■ SYNTHETIC QUESTIONS AND QUANTITATIVE PROBLEMS

1. Behavior itself is not inherited; what is inherited is genes. Genes direct the manufacture of proteins that are important in the formation of neural circuits that in turn underlie behavior. Some simple behavioral traits like color blindness or Huntington's disease are controlled by a single gene. More complex behavioral traits like schizophrenia or bipolar affective disorder are controlled by many genes acting in concert. In addition, behavior is shaped by a nongenetic component—the organism's interaction with the environment.

2. The lifetime risk of developing schizophrenia is strongly related to how close an individual is genetically related to a diagnosed schizophrenic. The highest risk is for identical twins, even if they were not raised in the same environment. There is progressively less risk for fraternal twins, siblings, nieces or nephews; the lowest risk is for people not related to a schizophrenic.

3. Humans have 46 chromosomes: 22 pairs of autosomes and one pair of sex chromosomes, either two Xs in females or an X and a Y in males. Since an individual receives one chromosome of each pair from each parent, sons always inherit their X chromosome from their mother. The genes for the red and green pigments used in color vision are on the X chromosome (i.e., they are X-linked), so that recessive mutations in those genes are usually expressed as red-green color blindness in males, who have only one copy, but not in females, who have two.

4. If two genes are located very close to one another, their phenotypes are likely to be inherited together. Thus, by tracing co-inheritance patterns of a disease and a number of phenotypes with known genetic locations (markers), one can map the approximate location of the gene for the disease. Markers used to locate the gene for Huntington's disease were mostly restriction fragment length polymorphisms, which are the result of differences in DNA sequence that produce or eliminate a cutting site for a particular restriction enzyme.

5. Cloned DNA from the gene is modified and introduced into mouse embryonic stem cells in culture by homologous recombination. The stem cells are then injected into a mouse embryo, which is implanted into a foster mother and allowed to come to term. This procedure produces a chimeric mouse that has some tissues that contain the modified gene and some that do not. If the modified gene has been incorporated into germ cells, animals that are homozygous for the mutation can be produced by selective breeding.

31

Sex and the Brain

Overview

A single gene determines the type of gonad in the fetus. Subsequent development of the fetus into a male or a female is controlled by hormones secreted from the gonads as well as by maternal hormones. The absence of male hormones leads to female development. The presence of male steroid hormones during a critical period around the time of birth produces permanent masculinization of the brain, resulting in a number of differences in the brains and behavior of male and female adults. These include differences in the size of particular brain nuclei, differences in growth of axons and dendrites, and hence neural circuitry, and differences in responsiveness of neurons in a variety of brain areas to sex hormones. These brain differences are associated with differences in reproductive behaviors (lordosis or mounting) as well as differences in cognitive abilities (spatial learning and verbal fluency).

Objectives

1. Understanding how gonad type is determined in early development.

2. Understanding how gonad sex hormones influence the subsequent development of male and female anatomy.

3. Understanding how sex hormones influence the development of the brain during a critical period in development.

4. Understanding the major anatomical and physiological differences in masculinized and feminized brains.

5. Understanding how the presence of sex hormones during the critical period influences adult reproductive behaviors.

6. Understanding cognitive differences between males and females during development and in adulthood.

■ COMPLETION PROBLEMS

1. Any characteristic that is different in males and females is called _____.

2. Individuals with Turner's syndrome have _____ Y chromosomes.

3. Testes secrete principally _____, ovaries _____.

4. Testosterone is converted to the female sex hormone _____.

5. Treatment of female monkey fetuses with _____ improves spatial learning when the animals become adults.

MULTIPLE CHOICE QUESTIONS

1. Persons with androgen insensitivity syndrome illustrate the following principle:

   A.   Functioning gonads are essential for gender identity.

   B.   Female external form and identity will develop if androgens do not have a functional receptor.

   C.   Male sexual behavior is independent of perinatal hormone secretion.

   D.   Absence of a functional androgen receptor results in mental retardation.

2. Persons with Turner's syndrome illustrate the following principle:

   A.   Functioning gonads are essential for gender identity.

   B.   Female form and sexual behavior can develop in the absence of gonadal steroids.

   C.   Male sexual behavior is independent of perinatal hormone secretion.

   D.   Absence of a sex chromosome is incompatible with life.

3. Appropriate steroid receptors are essential for the effectiveness of circulating hormones. In neurons these receptors

   A.   are transmembrane proteins.

   B.   use cyclic AMP as a second messenger.

   C.   are DNA binding proteins that alter transcription of specific proteins.

   D.   are identical for estrogen and testosterone.

4. Castration of a male rat immediately after birth has which of the following effects on sexual behavior?

   A. There is no effect on normal sexual behavior, as the castration occurred after the organization of the "male" brain was completed.

   B. Normal male sexual behavior will be present as long as testosterone can be aromatized to estradiol in the brain.

   C. Female sexual behaviors will occur if the male rat is exposed to estrogen and progesterone as an adult.

   D. There will be no sexual behavior regardless of adult hormonal treatment.

5. Analysis of cognitive functions in primates, including humans, has shown that there are cognitive differences related to age and gender. These include all of the following *except*:

   A. Boys tend to develop hemispheric specialization for tactile discrimination earlier than girls.

   B. Girls show a greater plasticity in transferring language function to the right hemisphere than do boys.

   C. Females test higher on mathematical reasoning.

   D. Males are more prone to developmental disorders associated with left hemisphere function, including developmental dyslexia, developmental aphasia, and infantile autism.

◼ TRUE/FALSE QUESTIONS
(If false, explain why)

1. Individuals with no gonads develop as females. _____

2. In adults, circulating steroid sex hormones do not affect sexual behavior. _____

3. Steroid sex hormones influence adult sexual behavior during a critical period around birth. _____

4. Female mice that develop between two male fetuses *in utero* are unusually aggressive as adults. _____

5. There are no detectable anatomical differences between male and female brains. _____

MATCHING QUESTIONS

1. Estrogen

2. Ovaries

3. Sry gene

4. Testes

5. Testosterone

A. androgens

B. estrogens

C. lordosis

D. mounting

E. testis-determining factor

SYNTHETIC QUESTIONS AND QUANTITATIVE PROBLEMS

1. Explain how gonad type is determined in early development.

2. Describe how gonadal hormones influence the subsequent development of male and female anatomy.

3. Sex hormones influence adult reproductive behaviors, such as lordosis and mounting, in different ways when they are present around birth or in adulthood. Briefly describe the different actions and some experimental results that illustrate these differences.

4. Explain why estrogens are even more effective than androgens in producing masculinization of the brain in genetic males, but genetic females are nonetheless not masculinized.

5. Describe differences in cerebral asymmetry in human males and females.

ANSWERS

■ COMPLETION PROBLEMS

1. sexual dimorphism

2. no

3. androgens; estrogens

4. estradiol

5. androgens

■ MULTIPLE CHOICE QUESTIONS

1. B.

2. B.

3. C.

4. C.

5. C.

■ TRUE/FALSE QUESTIONS

1. True

2. False. Sex hormones tend to activate sexual behavior in adults.

3. True

4. True

5. False. There are differences in the size of particular brain nuclei, as well as differences in the growth of axons and dendrites of particular types of neurons.

■ MATCHING QUESTIONS

1. C.

2. B.

3. E.

3. A.

4. D.

SYNTHETIC QUESTIONS AND QUANTITATIVE PROBLEMS

1. Gonad type (ovary or testis) is determined by a single gene, *sex-determining region of Y* (SRY), located on the short arm of the Y chromosome. The product of this gene, *testis determining factor* (TDF), causes the undifferentiated gonad to develop into a testis; in the absence of TDF the gonad becomes an ovary.

2. Fetal testes secrete two major hormones: testosterone and Müllerian duct-inhibiting substance (MIS). Testosterone masculinizes the sex organs and mammary gland rudiments. MIS causes resorption of tissue that would become the oviducts, uterus, cervix, and vagina. The absence of these two hormones results in the development of a female.

3. Exposure to specific sex hormones during a critical period around birth causes permanent changes in the nervous system that influence the type of adult behavior that is expressed. Sex hormones in adulthood have more of an activating function. For example, exposure of female rat pups to testosterone at birth (but not after postnatal day 10) results in adult animals with high levels of mounting behavior when treated with androgen, and low levels of lordosis when treated with estrogen. Similarly, castration of male rat pups at birth (but not after postnatal day 10) results in adult animals that show lordosis when treated with estrogen.

4. Intracellular enzymes in the target cells convert testosterone to the estrogen estradiol, which in turn causes masculinization by binding to nuclear receptors. In females (and males) the estrogen-binding protein alpha-fetoprotein in blood and cerebrospinal fluid protects the cells from circulating estrogen (but not from androgen).

5. In most humans the left hemisphere is specialized for language and the right hemisphere is specialized for nonverbal processes such as tactile recognition of three-dimensional objects. Boys show evidence of this hemispheric specialization as early as age 6, whereas girls do not show specialization until age 13. Correspondingly, damage to the left hemisphere has less effect on language in girls than in boys. This difference persists into adulthood, suggesting that the adult female brain is functionally less asymmetrical than the male brain.

32

Emotional States

Overview

Emotions have both a cognitive component, involving the cerebral cortex, and an autonomic component, involving the amygdala, hypothalamus, and brain stem. The James–Lange and Cannon–Bard theories proposed that the cognitive component follows the autonomic component as a result of input to the cortex from the periphery and hypothalamus. The hypothalamus maintains homeostasis of autonomic functions via its connections to the autonomic nervous system and the endocrine system. The autonomic nervous system is divided into the sympathetic division, which produces fight or flight reactions, and the parasympathetic division, which produces rest and digest reactions. The hypothalamus produces endocrine actions both directly by neurosecretion from the posterior pituitary and indirectly by secreting releasing hormones that act on the anterior pituitary.

Papez proposed that the cognitive and autonomic components of emotion affect each other reciprocally as a result of reciprocal connections between the cerebral cortex and hypothalamus through the limbic system, which includes the cingulate gyrus, hippocampus, amygdala and mammillary body. Of these, the amygdala plays a particularly prominent role. It receives sensory information from the thalamus and cortex and produces autonomic emotional responses (by projections to the hypothalamus and brain stem) and cognitive emotional responses (by projections to the cingulate gyrus and frontal cortex). Lesions of any of these structures or pathways produce characteristic changes in emotional responses.

Objectives

1. Understanding the James–Lange and Cannon–Bard theories of emotion.

2. Understanding the anatomy and function of the autonomic nervous system.

3. Understanding the direct and indirect endocrine functions of the hypothalamus and its relation to the pituitary.

4. Understanding the Papez theory of emotion.

5. Understanding the neural circuits of the limbic system.

6. Understanding the input and output connections of the amygdala.

7. Understanding the effects of lesions of different brain areas on emotional behavior.

◼ *COMPLETION PROBLEMS*

1. "Fight-or-flight" responses are controlled by the _____ division of the autonomic nervous system, whereas "rest and digest" responses are controlled by the _____ division.

2. The posterior lobe of the pituitary is called the _____, whereas the anterior lobe is called the _____.

3. Oxytonin and vasopressin are released by _____ neurons in the hypothalamus, whereas thyrotropin-releasing hormone and gonadotropin-releasing hormone are released by _____ neurons.

4. Klüver and Bucy found that bilateral removal of the _____ affects the emotionality of monkeys.

5. The _____ nuclei of the amygdala receive sensory input.

■ MULTIPLE CHOICE QUESTIONS

1. Normal emotions involve

    A. subcortical mechanisms exclusively.

    B. cortical (primarily limbic) structures exclusively.

    C. both subcortical and cortical structures.

    D. none of the above, since there is little evidence showing an involvement of either cortical or subcortical mechanisms.

2. Which of the following structures is part of the limbic system?

    A. Posterior thalamic nucleus.

    B. Raphe nuclei.

    C. PVN of the hypothalamus.

    D. Deep cerebellar nuclei.

    E. Cingulate gyrus.

3. Where do hypothalamic neurons release peptides?

    A. The anterior pituitary.

    B. The posterior pituitary.

    C. Both A and B.

    D. Neither A nor B.

4. Bioactive peptides are found prominently in what type of hypothalamic neuron?

    A. Magnocellular.

    B. Parvocellular.

    C. Both A and B.

    D. Neither A nor B.

5. Monkeys with bilateral removal of the temporal lobe are

   A.   tame.

   B.   unemotional.

   C.   highly oral.

   D.   highly sexual.

   E.   all of the above.

■ TRUE/FALSE QUESTIONS
(If false, explain why)

1. All of the structures of the limbic system are located in the brain stem. _____

2. All autonomic motor neurons are located outside the central nervous system. _____

3. Autonomic responses are usually not conscious. _____

4. Electrical stimulation of a single part of the hypothalamus produces a single autonomic response. _____

5. Lesions of the amygdala affect place conditioning. _____

■ MATCHING QUESTIONS

1. Increased heart rate

2. Resting heart rate

3. Release of vasopressin

4. Release of thyrotropin-releasing hormone

5. Fear conditioning

6. Emotional response to chronic pain

A. amygdala

B. anterior pituitary

C. parasympathetic nervous system

D. posterior pituitary

E. prefrontal cortex

F. sympathetic nervous system

■ SYNTHETIC QUESTIONS AND QUANTITATIVE PROBLEMS

1. Compare the James–Lange, Cannon–Bard, and Papez theories of emotion.

2. Draw a diagram (using arrows and boxes) illustrating the limbic system circuit proposed by Papez, and originally suggested as mediating aspects of emotional behavior (label the four main structures).

3. List several autonomic responses that occur during the emotion of fear and describe the anatomy of the effector system that controls these responses.

4. Describe the two ways in which activity of hypothalamic neurons can cause release of hormones from the pituitary.

5. Describe in general terms the inputs and outputs of the amygdala and their functional significance.

ANSWERS

COMPLETION PROBLEMS

1. sympathetic; parasympathetic

2. neurohypophysis; adenohypophysis

3. magnocellular; parvocellular

4. temporal lobe

5. basolateral

MULTIPLE CHOICE QUESTIONS

1. C.

2. E.

3. C.

3. C.

4. E.

TRUE/FALSE QUESTIONS

1. False. The limbic system includes *forebrain structures*.

2. True

3. True

4. False. It often produces a coordinated set of responses.

5. True

MATCHING QUESTIONS

1. F.

2. C.

3. D.

4. B.

5. A.

6. E.

SYNTHETIC QUESTIONS AND QUANTITATIVE PROBLEMS

1. James and Lange proposed that the cognitive component of emotion results from conscious perception of the peripheral, autonomic signs of emotion. Cannon and Bard proposed that the cognitive component of emotion results from input to the cerebral cortex from the hypothalamus, which also initiates the autonomic component. Papez proposed that the cognitive and autonomic components of emotion affect each other reciprocally, as a result of reciprocal connections between the cortex and hypothalamus.

2. Should show circuit going: from cingulate gyrus, to hippocampal formation, to hypothalamus (or mammillary body), to anterior thalamic nuclei, back to cingulate gyrus. See Figure 32–9 in the textbook, p. 607.

3. Increased heart rate, decreased salivation, increased respiration, sweating, pupillary constriction, urination, and defecation are all controlled by the sympathetic division of the autonomic nervous system. Motor neurons of the sympathetic system are located in autonomic ganglia and send axons to various smooth muscles and glands. Preganglionic neurons are located in the thoracic and lumbar spinal cord.

4. Magnocellular neurons send axons to the posterior pituitary, where they release peptides into the general circulation ("neurosecretion"). Parvocellular hypothalamic neurons release peptides ("releasing hormones") into the hypophyseal portal system, where they stimulate or inhibit secretions of hormones from the anterior pituitary gland.

5. The amygdala receives sensory information both from sensory cortex and from sensory nuclei in the thalamus. The input from the thalamus permits very rapid reactions to emotionally significant stimuli, whereas the input from the cortex permits finer discrimination of sensory stimuli. The amygdala sends projections to a wide variety of regions controlling different aspects of emotional response, including the hypothalamus and brain stem, which control autonomic responses, and the cerebral cortex, which is involved in the cognitive component of emotion.

33

Motivation

Overview

Motivation is an inferred internal state that is postulated to explain variability in basic behaviors related to survival, such as eating and drinking. Motivation or "drive" increases with deprivation, and directs, activates, and organizes behavior to help achieve homeostatic control of the internal environment. Thus, motivated behaviors can be thought of in terms of servocontrol mechanisms. This analogy is most directly applicable to control of body temperature: changes in temperature activate neurons in the hypothalamus that produce a variety of autonomic, endocrine, and skeletal responses to counteract those changes. Similarly, other neurons in the hypothalamus are involved in controlling feeding to maintain approximately constant body weight, or in controlling drinking to maintain tissue osmolarity and vascular fluid volume.

In addition to these physiological feedback mechanisms, behavior can also be affected by ecological constraints, anticipatory mechanisms, and hedonic (pleasure) factors. Insights into these different processes have come from studies in which animals work to receive electric stimulation or drug injection directly into the brain, rather than food or water. These studies suggest a prominent role for dopaminergic pathways in motivated behavior.

Objectives

1. Understanding the general features of motivation.

2. Understanding basic servocontrol theory and how it might explain simple motivation processes.

3. Understanding the physiological mechanisms of temperature regulation.

4. Understanding the internal variables and physiological mechanisms for the control of feeding and drinking.

5. Understanding the nonphysiological factors in the control of feeding and drinking.

6. Understanding experiments on self-administration of electric current or drugs to the brain, and the neural pathways thought to be involved.

■ COMPLETION PROBLEMS

1. The two main physiological variables that control drinking are _____ and _____.

2. Urges or impulses to action based on bodily needs are called _____.

3. External stimuli that are capable of driving behavior are called _____.

4. Injection of the peptide _____ into the hypothalamus causes voracious eating, particularly of carbohydrates.

5. Injection of the peptide _____ into the ventricles inhibits feeding.

6. The peptide _____ stimulates drinking.

MULTIPLE CHOICE QUESTIONS

1. In a servocontrol system the set point signal directly feeds into
   A. an integrator or error detector.
   B. the controlled system.
   C. the feedback detectors.
   D. the error signal.

2. The concept of set point
   A. applies only to temperature regulation.
   B. applies only to regulation of body weight.
   C. applies to both weight and temperature regulation.
   D. none of the above.

3. Lesions of the lateral hypothalamus result in
   A. decreased feeding.
   B. increased feeding.
   C. either increased or decreased feeding, depending on the size of the lesion.
   D. typically no effect on feeding.

4. Lesions of the anterior hypothalamus result in
   A. chronic depression of normal body temperature.
   B. chronic hyperthermia.
   C. swings between abnormally high and abnormally low body temperature.
   D. failure to maintain body temperature when challenged by cold environments.
   E. none of the above.

5. Based on what you know about regulation of drinking behavior, what would you expect would be the results of increasing blood volume (via transfusion) in a normal animal?

   A. Drinking will be stimulated.

   B. Drinking will be suppressed.

   C. There should be no effect on drinking.

   D. Drinking will be initially stimulated, then depressed.

   E. Drinking will be initially depressed, then stimulated.

6. Hedonic factors have an effect on feeding. What does this mean?

   A. Feeding behavior is dependent on the sex of the organism.

   B. Animals eat exclusively for the taste of a stimulus.

   C. Pleasure is one factor that regulates feeding.

   D. Feeding is not dependent on the level of deprivation.

   E. None of the above.

7. Under similar environmental conditions, individuals within a species

   A. have very similar body weight.

   B. have very similar daily energy expenditure.

   C. show a similar ratio of daily energy expenditure to metabolic body size (i.e., body weight raised to a power close to 0.7).

   D. all of the above.

   E. none of the above.

◼ *TRUE/FALSE QUESTIONS*
(If false, explain why)

1. Hypothalamic lesions can result in an animal *increasing* its body weight above its normal set point. _____

2. Hunger can be measured with electrophysiological recording devices. _____

3. Feedback about body temperature is provided by cells located in the hypothalamus and spinal cord. _____

4. Lesions of the hypothalamus can alter the set point for regulation of body weight. _____

5. Motivational states can be regulated only by tissue needs. _____

◼ *MATCHING PROBLEMS*

1. Decreased body temperature
2. Increased body temperature
3. Antipyretic response
4. Decreased feeding
5. Increased feeding
6. Circadian rhythm of feeding

A. anterior hypothalamus
B. lateral hypothalamus
C. medial hypothalamus
D. posterior hypothalamus
E. septal nuclei
F. suprachiasmatic nucleus

■ SYNTHETIC QUESTIONS AND QUANTITATIVE PROBLEMS

1. The concept of motivation has been compared to a flush toilet with a water storage tank. Explain this analogy and describe aspects of motivation that it does not address.

2. Using boxes and arrows, show the basic elements and connections of a servocontrol system.

3. Describe functional inputs and outputs of the hypothalamus involved in the regulation of temperature.

4. Briefly described several types of short-term physiological signals that act on the hypothalamus to help regulate the size of individual meals.

5. Describe electrical self-stimulation of the brain in behavioral experiments and what the results suggest about the role of dopamine in normal reinforcement and drug addiction.

ANSWERS

COMPLETION PROBLEMS

1. osmolarity; vascular fluid volume

2. drives

3. incentive stimuli

4. neuropeptide Y

5. cholecystokinin, neurotensin, calcitonin, or glucagon

6. angiotensin II

MULTIPLE CHOICE QUESTIONS

1. A.

2. C.

3. A.

4. B.

5. B.

6. C.

7. C.

TRUE/FALSE QUESTIONS

1. True

2. False. Hunger is inferred from behavior.

3. True

4. True

5. False. Motivational state is also influenced by anticipatory mechanisms and hedonic factors.

MATCHING PROBLEMS

1. A.

2. D.

3. E.

4. C.

5. B.

6. F.

SYNTHETIC QUESTIONS AND QUANTITATIVE PROBLEMS

1. Flushing the toilet corresponds to consummatory behavior triggered by an appropriate goal object. The level of water in the tank corresponds to the level of the drive for a particular type of behavior. The strength of a flush depends on the time since the last flush, corresponding to an increase in drive with increasing deprivation. This analogy does not reflect the idea that motivation directs and organizes behavior toward certain goals, or that it helps achieve homeostatic control of internal variables related to survival.

2. The drawing should include a set point signal feeding into a comparator, the output of which (the "error signal") feeds into controlling elements that alter the controlled system. Feedback detectors send a signal from the controlled system back to the comparator, where it subtracts from the setpoint signal (see Figure 33–1 in the textbook, p. 615).

3. Neurons in the hypothalamus change their firing in response to changes in the local temperature, and also in response to signals from temperature sensors in the periphery. The output of the hypothalamus can influence a variety of different types of effectors related to temperature, including autonomic, endocrine, nonvoluntary skeletal, and voluntary skeletal responses.

4. Chemical properties of food act in the mouth to stimulate feeding and in the gastrointestinal system and liver to inhibit feeding via afferent pathways to the hypothalamus. In addition, the hypothalamus has glucoreceptors that respond to blood glucose levels, and receptors for hormones that are released from the gut during a meal, such as cholecystokinin.

5. Electrical stimulation of the hypothalamus and associated structures can act as reinforcement in operant conditioning of animals, much like food or water. Brain stimulation differs from natural reinforcers, however, in that it does not depend on the drive state of the animal. Electrical stimulation in the hypothalamus is thought to activate nondopaminergic descending fibers in the medial forebrain bundle, which indirectly activate ascending dopaminergic fibers in the mesocorticolimbic pathway. Since cocaine and nicotine lower the threshold for electrical self-stimulation, and raise dopamine levels in the mesocorticolimbic pathway, this pathway may play a critical role in both normal reinforcement and drug addiction.

34

Language

Overview

Language is a distinctive form of communication that is much more highly developed in humans than in any other species. Several lines of evidence suggest that the capability for language is largely innate, which led Noam Chomsky to suggest that languages have a universal grammar that is determined by the structure of the brain. In the last century Wernicke found that damage to the left temporal lobe produces a deficit in comprehension of speech, while Broca found that damage to the left frontal lobe produces a deficit in speech production. Based on these observations, Wernicke and subsequently Geschwind proposed that processing of speech occurs in a series of steps in discrete regions of the cortex. Deficits in several other aspects of language, including emotional tone, reading, and writing, are also associated with abnormalities in specific areas of the brain.

Objectives

1. Understanding how language is distinctive from other forms of communication, including animal communication.

2. Understanding the evidence suggesting that the capability for language is largely innate.

3. Understanding the characteristic features of the three major types of aphasia (Wernicke's, Broca's, and conduction), and the brain areas that are damaged in each.

4. Understanding the Wernicke–Geschwind model of language processing and the weaknesses of the model.

5. Understanding the major characteristics of alexia, agraphia, and dyslexia, and the brain abnormalities associated with each.

■ COMPLETION PROBLEMS

1. In _____ aphasia verbal output is fluent but language comprehension is impaired, whereas in _____ aphasia verbal output is nonfluent and language comprehension is normal.

2. The smallest unit of sound that will affect the meaning of a word is a _____.

3. The rules for combining words to form phrases and sentences are called _____.

4. The pygmy chimpanzee Kanzi was able to comprehend language at the level of a _____ year-old human.

5. A motor impairment in speech articulation is called _____.

6. An acquired disruption of the ability to read is called _____.

7. A congenital disruption of the ability to read is called _____.

■ MULTIPLE CHOICE QUESTIONS

1. Aphasia is an acquired disorder of

    A.   reading.

    B.   speech.

    C.   thinking and feeling.

    D.   language.

    E.   perception.

2. Aphasia is caused by all of the following *except*

    A.   head injury.

    B.   brain tumor.

    C.   stroke.

    D.   Alzheimer's disease.

    E.   dysarthria.

3. Which of the following statements about aphasia is false?

    A.   Aphasias are commonly seen in patients with brain diseases.

    B.   Aphasias occur with stroke, dementia, and brain tumors.

    C.   Aphasias affect only right-handed individuals.

    D.   Aphasias can include impaired reading and writing.

    E.   Aphasias can result from injury to either the left or right hemisphere of the brain, but most often follow left hemisphere injury.

4. Which of the following descriptive phrases usually applies to Wernicke's aphasia?

    A.   Nonfluent.

    B.   Normal comprehension.

    C.   Difficulty repeating simple words or phrases.

    D.   Hemiparesis.

    E.   Normal reading.

5. In the syndrome of alexia without agraphia, or "pure word blindness," patients are unable to read but retain the ability to write. Which of these other signs is usually present?

   A. Hemiparesis.

   B. Confusion.

   C. Neologism.

   D. A lesion in the posterior corpus callosum

   E. A lesion in the left frontal operculum.

◼ *TRUE/FALSE QUESTIONS*
(If false, explain why)

1. Given appropriate training, animals such as chimpanzees can learn language comparably to humans. _____

2. In most humans the planum temporale in the right hemisphere is larger than that in the left. _____

3. Brain assymetries associated with language existed in *Homo erectus* as much as 500,000 years ago. _____

4. Brain assymetries associated with language exist *in utero*. _____

5. Dyslexic males generally have less than normal bilateral asymmetry in the planum temporale. _____

6. Dyslexic people generally have below-average I.Q. _____

MATCHING PROBLEMS

1. Broca's aphasia

2. Wernicke's aphasia

3. Conduction aphasia

4. Aprosodias

5. Alexia without agraphia

6. Alexia with agraphia

A. left frontal cortex

B. right frontal cortex

C. left occipital cortex

D. left parietal cortex

E. left parietal-temporal-occipital cortex

F. left temporal cortex

SYNTHETIC QUESTIONS AND QUANTITATIVE PROBLEMS

1. Describe four ways in which language is distinctive from all other forms of communication.

2. Describe two ways in which the development of language resembles development of vision, supporting the idea that the capability for language is largely an innate property of the brain.

3. List, in order, the cortical areas involved in repeating a printed word, according to the Wernicke–Geschwind model.

4. Describe four ways in which the Wernicke–Geschwind model is an oversimplification.

5. Describe two neuronal abnormalities associated with dyslexia.

ANSWERS

◼ COMPLETION PROBLEMS

1. Wernicke's; Broca's

2. phoneme

3. syntax

4. 2 to 3

5. dysarthria

6. alexia

7. dyslexia

◼ MULTIPLE CHOICE QUESTION

1. D.

2. E.

3. C.

4. C.

5. D.

◼ TRUE/FALSE QUESTIONS

1. False. Chimpanzees can learn language at the level of a 2 to 3-year-old human.

2. False. The left planum temporale is usually larger than the right.

3. True

4. True

5. True

6. False. They generally have normal I.Q.

◼ MATCHING PROBLEMS

1. A.

2. F.

3. D.

4. B.

5. C.

6. E.

■ SYNTHETIC QUESTIONS AND QUANTITATIVE PROBLEMS

1. (1) *Creativity.* We can readily generate and understand sentence we have never heard before. (2) *Form.* Languages use a limited number of elementary units that can be combined according to certain rules that constitute the structure or grammar of the language. (3) *Content.* Language can communicate abstractions and emotions as well as specific facts. (4) *Use.* Language is predominantly a means for social communication.

2. (1) At birth infants are able to distinguish a broad range of sounds. Children lose the ability to distinguish sounds that are not discriminated in the language they learn. (2) There is a critical period in development (roughly 2 years old to puberty) during which a language can be learned completely fluently. These two features of the development of language are similar to the development of the visual system, where ocular dominance columns do not develop properly without binocular experience during a critical period.

3. (1) Primary visual cortex, (2) higher-order visual cortex, (3) parietal-temporal-occipital association cortex (angular gyrus), (4) Wernicke's area, (5) parietal cortex (arcuate fasciculus), (6) Broca's area, (7) motor cortex.

4. (1) Lesions that produce the clinical syndromes are generally larger than the specific cortical areas of the model. (2) Subcortical regions are also involved in speech production. (3) Visual input may bypass Wernicke's area. (4) There may be separate pathways for recognizing or producing nonsense words.

5. (1) A smaller than normal planum temporale in the left hemisphere, with cytoarchitectonic abnormalities. (2) Slower than average processing in the fast-conducting components of the visual and auditory pathways.

35

Learning and Memory

Overview

Learning is the process by which animals acquire knowledge about the world, and memory is the retention of that knowledge over time. Clinical studies of patients with specific brain lesions indicate that there are two types of learning, explicit and implicit, that involve different brain areas. Explicit learning encodes information about autobiographical events and factual knowledge. Lesions of the medial temporal lobe, including the hippocampus, severely impair new explicit learning, although old explicit memories remain intact. It is therefore thought that the hippocampus is involved in processing newly learned information for a period of hours to weeks before it is stored elsewhere, perhaps in neocortex.

Implicit learning involves improvement in sensory or motor performance. Implicit learning can in turn be divided into nonassociative learning, such as habituation and sensitization, and associative learning, such as classical or operant conditioning. Implicit memories are thought to be encoded in the particular sensory and motor pathways involved in the learning task, including the amygdala and cerebellum. Both explicit and implicit memory have a short-term stage, which is susceptible to disruption by treatments such as electroconvulsive therapy, and a long-term stage, which is less susceptible.

Objectives

1. Understanding the symptoms of patients with damage to the medial temporal lobes.

2. Understanding the major features of explicit and implicit learning.

3. Understanding nonassociative and associative learning.

4. Understanding the basic operations of classical and operant conditioning and the biological constraints on conditioning.

5. Understanding why conditioning is thought to involve learning about predictive relations in the world.

6. Understanding which brain areas are thought to be involved in which aspects of learning.

7. Understanding the evidence indicating that memory has short-term and long-term stages.

■ COMPLETION PROBLEMS

1. Sensitization is a type of _____ learning, whereas classical conditioning is a type of _____ learning.

2. _____ is a decrease in responses to a repeated benign stimulus.

3. During classical conditioning a _____ generally occurs just after a _____.

4. During operant conditioning a _____ generally occurs just after a _____.

5. Selective memory loss for events that occurred before a trauma is called _____.

MULTIPLE CHOICE QUESTIONS

1. In operant conditioning an animal learns to

    A. associate its behavior with some environmental (reinforcing) event.

    B. associate a stimulus with poison-induced nausea.

    C. associate one stimulus (the conditioned stimulus) with another stimulus (the unconditioned stimulus).

    D. gradually cease responding to meaningless or unimportant stimuli.

    E. imitate the motor acts of another animal.

2. Brain trauma results in very substantial disruption of which type of memory?

    A. Recently acquired memories.

    B. Memories acquired five or more years previous to the trauma.

    C. Recent and remote memories, approximately to the same degree.

    D. Primarily implicit learning.

    E. Primarily memories of spatial location.

3. You view a one-legged kangaroo barging into the classroom. This will likely result in what type of learning?

    A. Implicit.

    B. Explicit.

    C. Operant.

    D. Sensitization.

    E. Imitative.

4. Bilateral damage to the hippocampus produces defects in what type of memory?

   A. Implicit.

   B. Sensitization.

   C. Both A and B.

   D. Neither A nor B.

5. Implicit memory typically

   A. requires repeated trials to build up.

   B. involves reconstruction of past events based on bits and pieces of remembered information.

   C. only includes classical conditioning.

■ *TRUE/FALSE QUESTIONS*
   (If false, explain why)

1. In operant conditioning, a CS (conditioned stimulus) is repeatedly paired with a UCS (unconditioned stimulus). _____

2. Explicit memories are always exactly like the original experience. _____

3. Explicit memory for a particular task, such as driving an automobile, can be superseded by implicit memory. _____

4. The "law of effect" states that behaviors that are rewarded tend to be repeated. _____

5. Computer models based on networks of neuron-like elements are able to simulate some cognitive processes but cannot generalize and do not function if any of the elements are damaged. _____

MATCHING PROBLEMS

1. Learning a telephone number   A. amygdala lesion

2. Eyeblink conditioning   B. cerebellar lesion

3. Conditioned fear   C. electroconvulsive therapy

4. Recent memory   D. hippocampal lesion

5. Long-term memory   E. protein synthesis inhibition

SYNTHETIC QUESTIONS AND QUANTITATIVE PROBLEMS

1. Compare the main features of explicit and implicit learning.

2. Describe the memory deficit of patients such as H.M., who had bilateral removal of the hippocampus and adjacent temporal lobes.

3. Describe the phenomenon of blocking, and explain what it illustrates about the nature of classical conditioning.

4. Describe food aversion conditioning and what it illustrates about biological constraints on learning.

ANSWERS

▓ COMPLETION PROBLEMS

1. nonassociative; associative

2. habituation

3. unconditioned stimulus; conditioned stimulus

4. reinforcer; operant response

5. retrograde amnesia

▓ MULTIPLE CHOICE QUESTIONS

1. A.

2. A.

3. B.

4. D.

5. A.

▪ *TRUE/FALSE QUESTIONS*

1. False. This happens in *classical conditioning*.

2. False. Explicit memories are often *reconstructed*.

3. True

4. True

5. False. They can generalize and tolerate damage to some elements.

▪ *MATCHING PROBLEMS*

1. D.

2. B.

3. A.

4. C.

5. E.

■ SYNTHETIC QUESTIONS AND QUANTITATIVE PROBLEMS

1. Explicit learning encodes information about autobiographical events and factual knowledge, can often be established in a single trial or experience, depends on conscious cognitive processes, and can be expressed in declarative statements. Implicit learning involves improvement in sensory or motor performance, accumulates slowly through repetition over many trials, does not depend on conscious cognitive processes, and ordinarily cannot be expressed in words.

2. H.M.'s old (e.g., childhood) memories are intact, and he is able to form new short-term memories. But he is unable to form new long-term memories. Moreover, this deficit is restricted to explicit learning, such as learning a number, a face, or spatial orientation. He has normal implicit learning, such as learning motor skills, classical conditioning, or perceptual priming.

3. A blocking experiment has two stages. During stage one a conditioned stimulus (CS_1) is paired with an unconditioned stimulus. During stage two, a compound conditioned stimulus ($CS_1 + CS_2$) is paired with the unconditioned stimulus. Generally, this procedure results in little conditioning of CS_2, even though CS_2 received many pairings with the US. This result illustrates that in classical conditioning animals do not simply learn about the temporal pairing of stimuli. Rather, they learn about the predictive value of the stimuli. In this experiment CS_2 does not improve the animal's ability to predict the US and therefore does not become conditioned.

4. If an animal becomes sick after eating a particular food, it learns not to eat that food again, even with a delay of hours between eating the food and becoming sick. Such learning does not occur if eating the food is followed by shock, or if hearing a tone is followed by sickness. These results illustrate that animals are predisposed to learn certain types of associations that have adaptive value.

36

Cellular Mechanisms of Learning and Memory

Overview

The mechanisms of learning and memory can be studied at the cellular level in a number of simple invertebrate and vertebrate preparations. Studies of invertebrates have shown that nonassociative implicit learning involves synaptic depression and facilitation. Short-term facilitation involves covalent modifications of preexisting proteins, whereas long-term facilitation involves gene regulation, synthesis of new proteins, and growth. Associative learning involves an activity-dependent enhancement of facilitation that can be explained by the properties of the adenylyl cyclase molecule.

Studies of mammals suggest that explicit learning involves long-term potentiation (LTP) in the hippocampus. LTP in the CA1 region of the hippocampus has associative (Hebbian) properties that can be explained by the properties of the NMDA receptor molecule.

These cellular mechanisms may also be involved in the modification of cortical somatotopic maps through experience, and in both the development and treatment of psychiatric disorders.

Objectives

1. Understanding the cellular mechanisms of habituation and sensitization of the gill-withdrawal reflex of *Aplysia*.

2. Understanding the mechanisms of short-term and long-term learning in *Aplysia*.

3. Understanding the mechanisms of nonassociative and associative learning in *Aplysia*.

4. Understanding the different properties and molecular mechanisms of long-term potentiation (LTP) in the CA1 and CA3 regions of the hippocampus.

5. Understanding the evidence suggesting that hippocampal LTP is important in spatial learning.

6. Understanding how somatotopic maps in the cortex can be modified by experience.

■ COMPLETION PROBLEMS

1. Habituation in *Aplysia* involves homosynaptic _____.

2. Sensitization in *Aplysia* involves heterosynaptic _____.

3. Induction of long-term potentiation in the CA1 region of hippocampus involves postsynaptic _____, but maintenance involves presynaptic _____, suggesting that there must be a _____ messenger.

4. The three cellular properties of LTP in the CA1 region of hippocampus that provide evidence for Hebb's postulate are _____.

5. Granule cells in the dentate gyrus send their axons through the _____ pathway to the CA3 region of hippocampus.

MULTIPLE CHOICE QUESTIONS

1. Which of the following mechanisms is involved in both short- and long-term facilitation in *Aplysia*?

    (1) Increased transmitter release.

    (2) Closure of K^+ channels.

    (3) Phosphorylation of existing proteins.

    (4) New protein synthesis.

    A.   1, 2, 3 correct.

    B.   1, 3 correct.

    C.   2, 4 correct.

    D.   4 correct.

    E.   All correct.

2. Which of the following mechanisms is involved in long-term, but not short-term, facilitation in *Aplysia*?

    (1) Increased transmitter release.

    (2) Closure of K^+ channels.

    (3) Phosphorylation of existing proteins.

    (4) New protein synthesis.

    A.   1, 2, 3 correct.

    B.   1, 3 correct.

    C.   2, 4 correct.

    D.   4 correct.

    E.   All correct.

3. Which of the following mechanisms are involved in both classical conditioning and sensitization in *Aplysia*?

    (1) Facilitation at sensory neuron-motor neuron synapses.

    (2) Increased transmitter release from the sensory neurons.

    (3) Increased cAMP levels in the sensory neurons.

    (4) A requirement for spike activity in the sensory neurons during training.

    A.   1, 2, 3 correct.

    B.   1, 3 correct.

    C.   2, 4 correct.

    D.   4 correct.

    E.   All correct.

4. Which of the following mechanisms are involved in classical conditioning, but not sensitization, in *Aplysia*?

    (1) Facilitation at sensory neuron-motor neuron synapses.

    (2) Increased transmitter release from the sensory neurons.

    (3) Increased cAMP levels in the sensory neurons.

    (4) A requirement for spike activity in the sensory neurons during training.

    A.   1, 2, 3 correct.

    B.   1, 3 correct.

    C.   2, 4 correct.

    D.   4 correct.

    E.   All correct.

5. Long-term potentiation in the CA3 region of hippocampus

    A.   is blocked by NMDA receptor antagonists.

    B.   has associative properties.

    C.   is blocked by injecting Ca^{2+} chelators into the postsynaptic neuron.

    D.   involves cAMP.

    E.   all of the above.

TRUE/FALSE QUESTIONS
(If false, explain why)

1. Habituation and sensitization in *Aplysia* involve changes in the same neurons that mediate the behavior. _____

2. Short-term sensitization in *Aplysia* involves increased sensitivity of receptors in the postsynaptic membrane. _____

3. Long-term sensitization in *Aplysia* involves an increase in the number of sensory neuron terminals. _____

4. Cellular mechanisms of nonassociative learning (sensitization) and associative learning (classical conditioning) in *Aplysia* are fundamentally different. _____

5. Somatotopic maps in somatic sensory cortex can be modified by normal experience in adults. _____

MATCHING PROBLEMS

1. Habituation

2. Sensitization

3. Long-term sensitization

4. Classical conditioning

5. Explicit learning

A. activity-dependent presynaptic facilitation

B. long-term potentiation

C. presynaptic facilitation

D. synaptic depression

E. synthesis of new proteins

■ SYNTHETIC QUESTIONS AND QUANTITATIVE PROBLEMS

1. Describe ways in which cellular mechanisms of short-term and long-term facilitation in *Aplysia* are similar, and ways in which they are different.

2. Both development of connections in the visual cortex and long-term potentiation in the hippocampus seem to require cooperative (synchronous) firing of more than one presynaptic neuron. Describe Hebbian synaptic plasticity and how it might explain this requirement for cooperativity.

3. What properties of the NMDA receptor-channel make it suitable for use in Hebbian synapses?

4. Describe experiments on mice with single gene knockouts that support a relationship between long-term potentiation and learning.

ANSWERS

◼ COMPLETION PROBLEMS

1. depression

2. facilitation

3. NMDA receptors, Ca^{2+} influx, or kinases

4. cooperativity; associativity; specificity

5. mossy fiber

◼ MULTIPLE CHOICE QUESTIONS

1. A.

2. D.

3. A.

4. D.

5. D.

■ TRUE/FALSE QUESTIONS

1. True

2. False. It involves increased *transmitter release.*

3. True

4. False. A mechanism of conditioning (activity-dependent presynaptic facilitation) is an elaboration of a mechanism of sensitization (presynaptic facilitation)

5. True

■ MATCHING PROBLEMS

1. D.

2. C.

3. E.

4. A.

5. B.

SYNTHETIC QUESTIONS AND QUANTITATIVE PROBLEMS

1. Both are produced by serotonin and cAMP and involve increased transmitter release, closure of K^+ channels, and phosphorylation of existing proteins. Only long-term facilitation involves persistent kinase activity, protein and RNA synthesis (and gene induction), and growth of new varicosities and active zones.

2. At Hebbian synapses coincident firing of both a pre- and postsynaptic neuron is required for strengthening of the synapse between the two cells. Cooperative (synchronous) firing of more than one presynaptic neuron is often necessary to cause firing of the postsynaptic neuron, as is required for Hebbian plasticity.

3. Opening of the NMDA receptor-channel requires both (1) binding of transmitter released from the presynaptic cell and (2) depolarization of the postsynaptic cell (which relieves Mg^{2+} block of the channel). These two conditions are produced when the pre- and postsynaptic neurons fire together, as is required for Hebbian plasticity at the synapse between the two cells.

4. Mice with knockouts of either the α subunit of calcium/calmodulin-dependent protein kinase or *fyn* tyrosine kinase have absent or reduced LTP, and reduced spatial learning in a water maze where they have to find a submerged platform. By contrast, their learning is normal in simple visual discrimination tasks.

Current Flow in Neurons

John Koester

Overview

The basic principles of electrical circuit theory are reviewed here. Familiarity with this material is important for understanding the equivalent circuit model of the neuron developed in Chapters 8–12. This Appendix is divided into three parts:

1. The definition of basic electrical parameters.
2. A set of rules for elementary circuit analysis.
3. A description of current flow in circuits with capacitance.

Definition of Electrical Parameters

Potential Difference (V or E)

Electrical charges exert an electrostatic force on other charges: like charges repel, opposite charges attract. As the distance between two charges increases, the force that is exerted decreases. *Work* is done when two charges that initially are separated are brought together: *negative work* is done if their polarities are opposite, and *positive work* if they are the same. The greater the values of the charges and the greater their initial separation, the greater the work that is done (work = $\int_r^0 f(r)\, dr$, where f is electrostatic force and r is the initial distance between the two charges). Potential difference is a measure of this work. The potential difference between two points is the work that must be done to move a unit of positive charge (1 coulomb), from one point to the other, i.e., it is the potential energy of the charge. One volt (V) is the energy required to move 1 coulomb a distance of 1 meter against a force of 1 newton.

Current (I)

A potential difference exists within a system whenever positive and negative charges are separated. Charge separation may be generated by a chemical reaction (as in a battery) or by diffusion between two electrolyte solutions with different ion concentrations across a permeability-selective barrier, such as a cell membrane. If a region of charge separation exists within a conducting medium, then charges move between the areas of potential difference: positive charges are attracted to the region with a more negative potential, and negative charges go to the regions of positive potential. The resulting movement of charges is current flow, which is defined as the net movement of positive charge per unit time. In metallic conductors current is carried by electrons, which move in the opposite direction of current flow. In nerve and muscle cells current is carried by positive and negative ions in solution. One ampere (A) of current represents the movement of 1 coulomb (of charge) per second.

Conductance (g)

Any object through which electrical charges can flow is called a conductor. The unit of electrical conductance is the siemen (S). According to Ohm's law the current that flows through a conductor is directly proportional to the potential difference imposed across it:*

$$I = V \times g$$

As charge carriers move through a conductor, some of their potential energy is lost; the lost energy is converted into thermal energy due to the frictional interactions of the charge carriers with the conducting medium.

Each type of material has an intrinsic property called *conductivity* (σ), which is determined by its molecular structure. Metallic conductors have very high conductivities, which means that they conduct electricity extremely well; aqueous solutions with high ionized salt concentrations have somewhat lower values of σ; and lipids have very low conductivities—they are poor conductors of electricity and are therefore good insulators. The conductance of an object is proportional to σ times its cross-

---

*This formula for describing current flow is analogous to other formulas describing flow, e.g., bulk flow of a liquid due to hydrostatic pressure, flow of a solute in response to a concentration gradient, or flow of heat in response to a temperature gradient. In each case flow is proportional to the product of a driving force times a conductance factor.

sectional area, divided by its length:

$$g = (\sigma) \times \frac{\text{Area}}{\text{Length}}$$

The length dimension is defined as the direction along which one measures conductance (between *a* and *b*):

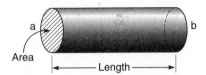

For example, the conductance measured across a piece of cell membrane is less if its length (thickness) is increased, e.g., by myelination. The conductance of a large area of membrane is greater than that of a small area of membrane.

Electrical resistance (R) is the reciprocal of conductance, and is a measure of the resistance provided by an object to current flow. Resistance is measured in ohms (Ω):

$$1 \text{ ohm} = (1 \text{ siemen})^{-1}.$$

Capacitance (C)

A capacitor consists of two conducting plates separated by an insulating layer. The fundamental property of a capacitor is its ability to store charges of opposite sign: positive charge on one plate, negative on the other.

A capacitor made up of two parallel plates with its two conducting surfaces separated by an insulator (an air gap) is shown in Figure A–1A, part 1. There is a net excess of positive charges on plate *x*, and an equal number of excess negative charges on plate *y*, resulting in a potential difference between the two plates. One can measure this potential difference by determining how much work is required to move a positive "test" charge from the surface of *y* to that of *x*. Initially, when the test charge is at *y*, it is attracted by the negative charges on *y*, and repelled less strongly by the more distant positive charges on *x*. The result of these electrostatic interactions is a force *f* that opposes the movement of the test charge from *y* to *x*. As the test charge is moved to the left across the gap the attraction by the negative charges on *y* diminishes, but the repulsion by the positive charges on *x* increases, with the result that the net electrostatic force exerted on the test charge is constant everywhere between *x* and *y* (Figure A–1A, part 2). Work (*W*) is force times the distance (*D*) over which the force is exerted:

$$W = f \times D.$$

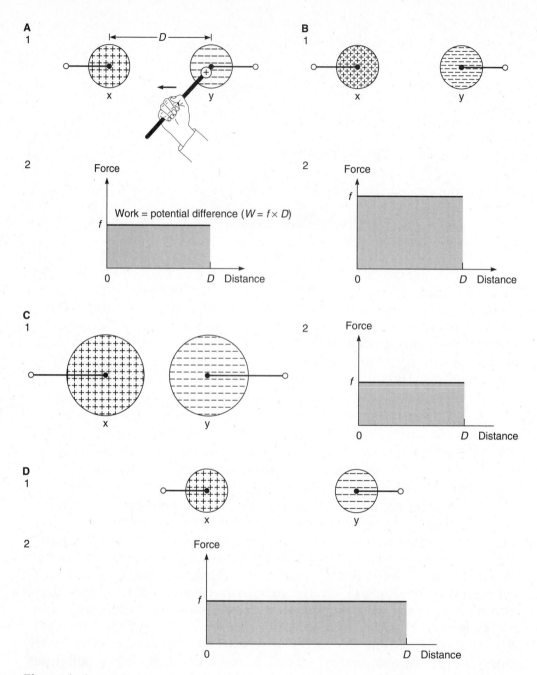

Figure A–1.

The factors that affect the potential difference between two plates of a capacitor.

 A. As a test charge is moved between two charged plates (1), it must overcome a force (2). The work done against this force is the potential difference between the two plates.

 B. Increasing the charge density (1) increases the potential difference (2).

 C. Increasing the area of the plates (1) increases the number of charges required to produce a given potential difference (2).

 D. Increasing the distance between the two plates (1) increases the potential difference between them (2).

Therefore, it is simple to calculate the work done in moving the test charge from one side of the capacitor to the other. It is the shaded area under the curve in Figure A–1A, part 2. This work is equal to the difference in electrical potential energy, or potential difference, between *x* and *y*.

Capacitance is measured in farads (F). The greater the density of charges on the capacitor plates, the greater the force acting on the test charge, and the greater is the resulting potential difference across the capacitor (Figure A–1B). Thus, for a given capacitor, there is a linear relationship between the amount of charge (*Q*) stored on its plates and the potential difference (*V*) across it:

$$Q \text{ (coulombs)} = C \text{ (farads)} \times V \text{ (volts)} \tag{A–1}$$

where the capacitance, *C*, is a constant.

The capacitance of a parallel-plate capacitor is determined by two features of its geometry: the area (*A*) of the two plates and the distance (*D*) between them. Increasing the area of the plates increases capacitance, because a greater amount of charge must be deposited on each side to produce the same charge density, which is what determines the force *f* acting on the test charge (Figure A–1A and C). Increasing the distance *D* between the plates does not change the force acting on the test charge, but it does increase the work that must be done to move it from one side of the capacitor to the other (Figures A–1A and D). Therefore, for a given charge separation between the two plates, the potential difference between them is proportional to the distance. Put another way, the greater the distance the smaller the amount of charge that must be deposited on the plates to produce a given potential difference, and therefore the smaller the capacitance (Equation A–1). These geometrical determinants of capacitance can be summarized by the equation:

$$C \, \alpha \, \frac{A}{D}.$$

As shown in Equation A–1, the separation of positive and negative charges on the two plates of a capacitor results in a potential difference between them. Conversely, the potential difference across a capacitor is determined by the excess of positive and negative charges on its plates. In order for the potential across a capacitor to change, the amount of electrical charges stored on the two conducting plates must change first.

Rules for Circuit Analysis

A few basic relationships that are used for circuit analysis are listed below. Familiarity with these rules will help in understanding the electric circuit examples that follow.

Conductance

The symbol for a conductor (or resistor) is:

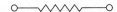

A variable conductor is represented this way:

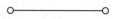

A pathway with infinite conductance (zero resistance) is called a short circuit, and is represented by a straight line:

Conductances in parallel add:

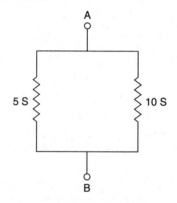

Conductances in series add reciprocally:

$$\frac{1}{g_{AB}} = \frac{1}{5} + \frac{1}{10} = \frac{3}{10}$$

$$g_{AB} = 3.3 \text{ S.}$$

Resistances in series add, while resistances in parallel add reciprocally.

Current

An *arrow* denotes the direction of current flow (net movement of positive charge).

Ohm's law is

$$I = Vg = \frac{V}{R}.$$

When current flows through a conductor, the end that the current enters is positive with respect to the end that it leaves:

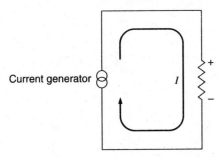

The algebraic sum of all currents entering or leaving a junction is zero (we arbitrarily define current approaching a junction as positive, and current leaving a junction as negative). In the following circuit

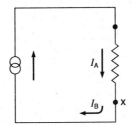

the currents for junction x are

$$I_A = +5 \text{ A}$$
$$I_B = -5 \text{ A}$$
$$I_A + I_B = 0.$$

In the following circuit

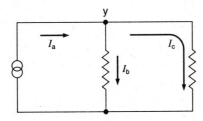

the currents for junction y are

$$I_a = +3 \text{ A}$$
$$I_b = -2 \text{ A}$$
$$I_c = -1 \text{ A}$$
$$I_a + I_b + I_c = 0.$$

Current follows the path of greatest conductance (least resistance). For conductance pathways in parallel, the current through each path is proportional to its conductance value divided by the total conductance of the parallel combination:

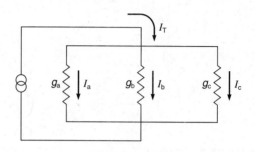

$$I_T = 10 \text{ A}$$
$$g_a = 3 \text{ S}$$
$$g_b = 2 \text{ S}$$
$$g_c = 5 \text{ S}$$

$$I_a = I_T \frac{g_a}{g_a + g_b + g_c} = 3 \text{ A}$$

$$I_b = I_T \frac{g_b}{g_a + g_b + g_c} = 2 \text{ A}$$

$$I_c = I_T \frac{g_c}{g_a + g_b + g_c} = 5 \text{ A}.$$

Capacitance

The symbol for a capacitor is:

The potential difference across a capacitor is proportional to the charge stored on its plates:

$$V_C = \frac{Q}{C}.$$

Potential Difference

The symbol for a battery, or electromotive force, is often abbreviated by the symbol *E*:

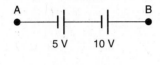

E

The positive pole is always represented by the longer bar.

Batteries in series add algebraically, so attention must be paid to their polarities. If their polarities are the same, their absolute values add:

A   B

5 V   10 V

$$V_{AB} = -15 \text{ V.}$$

If their polarities are opposite, they subtract:

A   B

5 V   10 V

$$V_{AB} = -5 \text{ V.}$$

The convention used here for potential difference is that $V_{AB} = (V_A - V_B)$.

A battery drives a current around the circuit from its positive to its negative terminal:

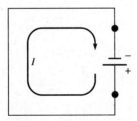

For purposes of calculating the total resistance of a circuit the internal resistance of a battery is set at zero.

The potential differences across parallel branches of a circuit are equal:

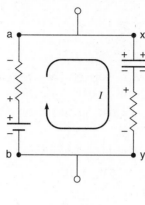

$$V_{ab} = V_{xy}.$$

As one goes around a closed loop in a circuit, the algebraic sum of all the potential differences is zero:

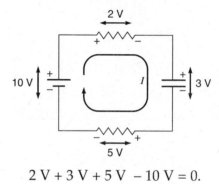

$$2\text{ V} + 3\text{ V} + 5\text{ V} - 10\text{ V} = 0.$$

Current Flow in Circuits with Capacitance

Circuits that have capacitive elements are much more complex than those that have only batteries and conductors. This complexity arises because current flow varies with time in capacitive circuits. The time dependence of the changes in current and voltage in capacitive circuits is illustrated qualitatively in the following three examples.

Capacitive Circuit

Capacitive current does not actually flow across the insulating gap in a capacitor; rather it results in a build-up of positive and negative charges on the capacitor plates.

However, we can measure a current flowing into and out of the terminals of a capacitor. Consider the circuit shown in Figure A–2A. When switch S is closed (Figure A–2B), a net positive charge is moved by the battery E onto plate a, and an equal amount of net positive charge is withdrawn from plate b. The result is current flowing counterclockwise in the circuit. Since the charges that carry this current flow into or out of the terminals of a capacitor, building up an excess of plus and minus charges on its plates, it is called a *capacitive current* (I_c). Because there is no resistance in this circuit, the battery E can generate a very large amplitude of current, which will charge the capacitance to a value $Q = E \times C$ in an infinitessimally short period of time (Figure A–2D).

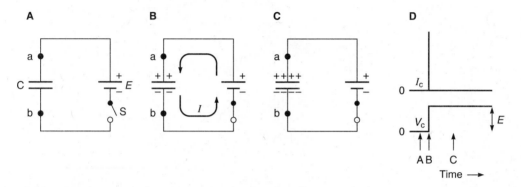

Figure A–2. Time course of charging a capacitor.
    A. Circuit before switch (S) is closed.
    B. Immediately after the switch is closed.
    C. After the capacitor has become fully charged.
    D. Time course of changes in I_c and V_c in response to closing of switch.

Circuit with Resistor and Capacitor in Series

Now consider what happens if a resistor is added in series with the capacitor in the circuit shown in Figure A–3A. The maximum current that can be generated when switch S is closed (Figure A–3B) is now limited by Ohm's law ($I = V/R$). Therefore, the capacitor charges more slowly. When the potential across the capacitor has finally reached the value $V_c = Q/C = E$ (Figure A–3C), there is no longer a difference in potential around the loop; i.e., the battery voltage (E) is equal and opposite to the voltage across the capacitor, V_c. The two thus cancel out, and there is no source of potential difference left to drive a current around the loop. Immediately after the switch is closed the potential difference is greatest, so current flow is at a maximum. As the capacitor begins to charge, however, the net potential difference ($V_c + E$) available to drive a current becomes smaller, so that current flow is reduced . The result is that an exponential change in voltage and in current flow occurs across the resistor and the capacitor. Note that in this circuit resistive current must equal capacitative current at all times (see Rules for Circuit Analysis, above).

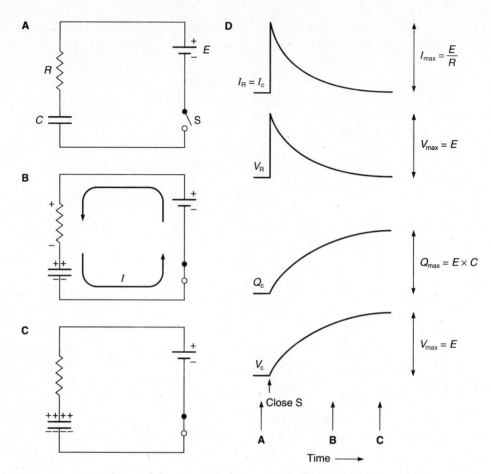

Figure A–3. Time course of charging a capacitor in series with a resistor, from a constant voltage source (E).
   A. Circuit before the switch (S) is closed.
   B. Shortly after switch is closed.
   C. After capacitor has settled at its new potential.
   D. Time course of current flow, of the increase in charge deposited on the capacitor, and of the increased potential differences across the resistor and the capacitor.

Circuit with Resistor and Capacitor in Parallel

Consider now what happens if we place a parallel resistor and capacitor combination in series with a constant current generator that generates a current I_T (Figure A–4). When switch S is closed (Figure A–4B), current starts to flow around the loop. Initially, in the first instant of time after the current flow begins, all of the current flows into the capacitor, i.e., $I_T = I_c$. However, as charge builds up on the plates of the capacitor, a potential difference V_c is generated across it. Since the resistor and capacitor are in parallel, the potential across them must be equal; thus part of the total current begins to flow through the resistor, such that $I_R R = V_R = V_c$. As less and less current flows into the capacitor, its rate of charging will become slower; this accounts for the exponential shape of the curve of voltage versus time. Eventually, a plateau is reached at which the voltage no longer changes. When this occurs, all of the current flows through the resistor, and $V_c = V_R = I_T R$.

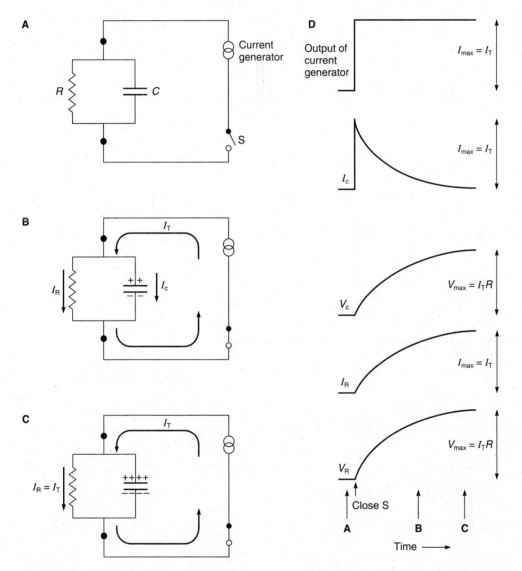

Figure A–4. Time course of charging a capacitor in parallel with a resistor, from a constant current source.

A. Circuit before switch (S) is closed.

B. Shortly after switch is closed.

C. After charge deposited on the capacitor has reached its final value.

D. Time course of changes in I_c, V_c, I_R, and V_R in response to closing of the switch.